Gianni Belcaro is a researcher at the Cardiovascular Institute of Chieti University, Italy, a Research Fellow in Vascular Surgery at the Irvine Cardiovascular Laboratory, St Mary's Hospital, London, and Director of the Vascular and Angiology Surgical Centre, Pescara, Italy. He is the author of *Laser Doppler, Vascular Screening* and *Venous Disorders: A Manual of Diagnosis and Treatment*. He has also published several papers on the subject.

Andrew N. Nicolaides, MS, FRCS, FRCSE, is Professor of Vascular Surgery, Honorary Consultant, and Director of the Irvine Laboratory for Cardiovascular Investigation, St Mary's Hospital Medical School, London. He is a member of the Vascular Society of Great Britain. His publications include *Thromboembolism Aetiology: Advances in Prevention and Management* (1975) and *The Investigation of Vascular Disorders* (1981), and a number of papers on aetiology, prevention and management of postoperative deep venous thrombosis and noninvasive cardiovascular investigation.

Gerard Stansby is Senior Lecturer and Honorary Consultant Surgeon at the Academic Surgical and Vascular Units, Imperial College School of Medicine, St Mary's Hospital, London. He is the author of over 50 academic articles.

The Venous Clinic

Diagnosis, Prevention, Investigations, Conservative and
Medical Treatment, Sclerotherapy and Surgery

Gianni Belcaro

Cardiovascular Institute, Chieti University, Italy,

Angiology & Vascular Surgery, Pierangeli Clinic, Pescara, Italy,

Irvine Laboratory for Cardiovascular Investigation and Research,
Department of Vascular Surgery, Division of Surgery, Anaesthetics and Intensive Care,
Imperial College and St Mary's Hospital, London, U.K.

Andrew N. Nicolaides

Irvine Laboratory for Cardiovascular Investigation and Research,
Department of Vascular Surgery, Division of Surgery, Anaesthetics and Intensive Care,
Imperial College and St Mary's Hospital, London, U.K.

Gerard Stansby

Division of Surgery, Anaesthetics and Intensive Care,
Imperial College, London, U.K.

In collaboration with:

G.B. Agus, A. Barsotti, M.R. Cesarone, D. Christopoulos, M.T. De Sanctis, S. Dhanjil, B. Eklof,
C. Fisher, G. Geroulakos, G. Gizzi, G. Goren, M. Griffin, D.T.A. Hardman, M. Herny, R. Hull,
L. Incandela, N. Labropoulos, A. Ledda, G. Laurora, M. Leon, A. Lennox, M. Malouf, G. Pineo,
G. Ramaswami, A. Ricci, O. Thulesius, J. Vale, S. Vasdekis, M. Veller,
R. Venniker, A. Zukoski and L.P. Willows

Imperial College Press

CP

Published by

Imperial College Press
203 Electrical Engineering Building
Imperial College
London SW7 2BT

Distributed by

World Scientific Publishing Co. Pte. Ltd.
P O Box 128, Farrer Road, Singapore 912805
USA office: Suite 1B, 1060 Main Street, River Edge, NJ 07661
UK office: 57 Shelton Street, Covent Garden, London WC2H 9HE

British Library Cataloguing-in-Publication Data
A catalogue record for this book is available from the British Library.

THE VENOUS CLINIC
Diagnosis, Prevention, Investigations, Conservative and Medical Treatment, Sclerotherapy and Surgery

ISBN 1-86094-051-X

Printed in Singapore.

Dedicated to Philip Sager and Alfred Bollinger.

CONTENTS

The Venous Clinic

PREFACE

That veins can cause disease has been known since classical times. However, our understanding of exactly how abnormalities of the venous system cause pathology has increased enormously in the last two decades. In line with this has come an expansion in the therapeutic modalities available along with inevitable controversies as to how they should be used. *The Venous Clinic* aims to cover in a relatively small volume all the wide-ranging conditions which have an abnormality of the venous system as their cause, and to outline strategies and principles of investigation and treatment. We hope it will appeal to a wide range of readers in different disciplines, including surgeons and physicians, nurses, medical technologists and those involved in venous research.

Venous disease, considered collectively, imposes an enormous burden on the health resources of most developed countries. Venous ulceration alone will be experienced by approximately 1% of all adults, and pulmonary embolism remains the major cause of death after elective surgery in young patients. Such facts would seem to justify the allocation of resources to the study of venous disease. Unfortunately, in most countries venous disorders have not traditionally received the focused attention that they deserve. Perhaps this is because these diseases often cross what would be considered the usual boundaries in medical specialisation and research. Now, however, phlebology is emerging as a valid and appropriate subspeciality, with its own research journals, meetings and areas of practice. This development is more advanced in some countries than in others, but considered overall it is a rapidly growing movement. It seems beyond debate that, armed with a special interest, knowledge and understanding of the mechanisms of venous disease, phlebologists will be able to provide the best and most appropriate standard of care in many instances or offer advice on investigation and treatment to their colleagues in other specialities. Perhaps more important, this may lead to more and better research into venous disease and its treatment. We believe that this book will support that philosophy and hopefully, in some small way, lead to a greater appreciation of the problems suffered by patients with venous disorders.

G. Stansby
G. Belcaro
A. N. Nicolaides

INTRODUCTION

The spectrum of venous diseases is large and much of the population is affected. Is it possible to screen patients with venous diseases and control the problem before it becomes symptomatic and expensive?

A positive answer comes from the experience of prevention of deep venous thrombosis (DVT) and pulmonary embolism (PE), which may be controlled and greatly reduced by preventive measures. However, it would also be important to know if it is possible to slow down the progression of venous insufficiency.

In this introduction we mainly consider the following problems:

- The *epidemiology* and *screening* of venous diseases;
- The evaluation of progression and of the efficacy of therapeutic measures by *quality of life assessment*;
- The correlation between some dietary factors (in particular, *"accessory" food elements* such as olive oil, fibres, berries and roots) and the incidence of venous diseases.

It is possible that these neglected aspects of venous disorders may be crucial in planning the best, most effective preventive measures and treatments to control a constellation of diseases affecting a large number of people with an otherwise normal life.

Epidemiology and Costs of Venous Diseases

Venous diseases (particularly chronic venous insufficiency and venous thromboembolism) are among the commonest problems in medicine. The precise distribution of venous diseases is largely unknown, as no prospective studies analysing a whole population, using noninvasive diagnostic technology (to define incompetence and/or obstruction), are available. In all developed countries varicose veins are a common problem and in European surgical wards some 30% of the nonmedical staff's time may be spent on chronic treatment of venous ulceration. Some 1% of men and 4–5% of women in Europe may have clinical venous problems. However, most statistical data result only from referrals to medical services. Therefore these figures are only partially related to the real incidence of venous diseases in the population as a whole.

Ideally only a population study including the whole population (or a defined *quota sampling*) may reveal the true prevalence of venous diseases including clinical and subclinical disease (for which there is no referral to medical services). A full knowledge of the prevalence of subclinical disease may give us an estimate of costs when the disease becomes symptomatic. A disease such as chronic venous insufficiency is ideal for screening, for several reasons:

(1) The prevalence in the population is high, possibly some 10% (there is no point in screening, or it is not cost-effective to screen, a population for a rare disease);

(2) The long time needed for subclinical problems (10–30 years) to progress to the clinical phase in most subjects. This long subclinical period of time is theoretically useful for avoiding the passage to clinical disease by secondary preventive measures;

(3) We have reliable and relatively low cost methods for evaluating venous problems (noninvasive investigations in venous disorders are very cost-effective in revealing the extent, degree and level of venous reflux or obstruction or both).

Finally, the distribution, awareness and level of tolerance for subclinical and clinical venous diseases — such as venous insufficiency, which is not life-threatening — are extremely variable among populations, from a zero level where nutritional and basic health problems are relevant (i.e. Third World countries) to extreme, almost paranoid, attention to even minor cosmetic problems in populations (or in population strata) with high standards of living and nothing better (or worse) to fear or to think about.

It is therefore important to evaluate the distribution of venous diseases in screening a population sample in full (or at least analysing a proportional sample representing the population distribution).

The San Valentino Vascular Screening Project

In July 1994 the San Valentino project was launched. An institute including a vascular laboratory was placed in the village of San Valentino (Central Italy, altitude 500 m, population about 2000). The *main aim of the study* was to evaluate the prevalence of early, subclinical atherosclerosis in the whole population. A second project was initiated with the *aim of evaluating the prevalence of venous diseases* in a homogeneous population (one single valley; low level of emigration and immigration in the previous 30 years). The *third part of the project was the evaluation of the progression of both arterial and venous diseases for a period of 10 years*. The clinical history was recorded and subjects were clinically examined (in the standing and the supine position). Leg circumferences were measured with a tape (calf and thigh). An ATL duplex scanner was used for the ultrasound evaluation. The noninvasive investigation methods used in the project are described in detail in Chapter 2. The clinical or subclinical patterns associated with venous diseases due to incompetence were classified according to the scheme presented in Table 1. The population examined at the end of 1996 included 746 subjects without arterial disease (379 females; mean age 46.3±7; range 8–94). The per cent distribution of venous diseases in this population is shown in Table 1. There was a trend for all venous diseases to increase with increasing age. The trend age/disease distribution was significantly higher for lipodermatosclerosis and ulceration. In total, 8.6% of the populations had at the time of the examination (or in their medical history) a clinically relevant venous problem. In some 3% within this group these problems were severe (they had been treated or were under treatment or had required hospital admission). In a further 2.8% the venous problem was less severe (not requiring treatment) or subclinical.

The use of medical products and treatments in these patients is indicated in Table 2. The average cost per patient for a year's treatment was 850 ECU, including hospital costs, lost days of work and medical products. Some 45% of these costs had been charged to the community services and hospitals (the health community) and the rest had been directly charged to the patients. We were able to (*arbitrarily*) calculate that more than 50% of the services, treatments and products used had been either inappropriate or ineffective. Considering that venous diseases are usually chronic, the community costs make these diseases a major heath care problem. Inefficiency, lack of

The Venous Clinic

Table 1. Clinical and subclinical venous patterns. The clinical or subclinical patterns associated with venous diseases of the lower limbs were classified according to the following scheme. The per cent of the population with each venous problem is shown. In 5.5% of the subjects more than one problem was present (i.e. teleangectasias and varicose veins).

Category	%
1. Teleangectasias	8
2. Varicose veins (no signs/symptoms or complications)	6
3. Varicose veins with mild initial complications (skin changes)	2
4. Severe superficial and/or deep incompetence (including chronic veins and severe complications, i.e. thrombophlebitis, bleeding, skin changes)	3.3
5. Chronic venous hypertension	2
6. Small ($< 1 cm^2$), initial (first) ulcerations	2
7. Severe, recurrent ulcerations with infection	1
8. Previous DVT (history only)	4
(documented)	1
9. Previous PE (history only)	<1
(documented)	0.2
10. Thrombophlebitis (history only)	8
(documented)	2.3

Table 2. Products used for the treatment of venous problems and per cent of patients with venous disease using them acutely (AC: once–twice) or chronically (CH: continuously for more than three months). More than one treatment was or has been used by some 9% of patients.

Products used for treatment	%	
	AC	CH
1. OTC products (or any treatment not requiring prescription)	18	7
2. Specialized drug (for venous diseases)	21	12
3. Compression	24	11
4. Surgery (any type of surgical treatment)	12	–
5. Sclerotherapy	9	3
6. Combined treatments (i.e. sclerotherapy and surgery)	9	8
7. Alternative treatments (herbal products etc.)	10	3

prevention and differences of standards possibly double the costs of venous diseases.

In conclusion, many of the population are affected by clinical venous problems and subclinical problems, which results in major costs for the health services of developed countries.

Whether screening of the youngest part of the population for venous problems before they become clinically relevant (and expensive) can be effective in reducing costs and controlling the evolution of many venous diseases is still to be evaluated. It is possible that in many subjects with early venous disease the control of progression and evolution to clinical stages may be obtained with simple preventive methods. Knowing correctly the sites and degree of incompetence, it is possible to suggest an *evolution controlling plan* using the several methods available (sclerotherapy, selective surgery, compression or medical treatment).

Quality of Life and Venous Diseases

Attempts to quantitatively evaluate venous diseases, their progression and the effects of treatment are a major problem in the venous clinic. The evaluation of ambulatory venous pressure (AVP) or air plethysmography (APG) parameters is useful for quantifying and evaluating the effects of treatment in groups of subjects but is complicated and time-consuming and does not always reflect the point of view of the single patient. From a patient's point of view the *quality of life (QOL)*, or its deterioration associated with the venous problem, is the most important criterion to consider. What is the point of changing AVP when the patient does not change his standard of life (i.e. requiring less medical consultation time, less cost for taking care of the problem and a more active life)? For a patient it is more important to be able to shop or to walk and buy a paper without help or difficulty than to undergo a purely physiological change (i.e. in venous pressure).

For a list of ten medical outcome QOL items (Table 3) an arbitrary quality-of-life score concerning venous problems may be considered. The total score varies between 0 and 100 (100 indicates a 100% fit subject). The decrease in the score indicates a deterioration in the patient's life due to any venous disease. If we consider a group of symptomatic subjects (89) with superficial

The Venous Clinic

Table 3. Medical outcome in venous diseases: quality of life score.

1. Mobility	0 ➔ 10
2. Pain	
3. Swelling	
4. Subjective symptoms	
5. Objective signs	
6. Independence	
7. Working life	
8. Social life	
9. Cosmetic aspect	
10. Costs (in time and money)	

Total   0–100
100 = 100% fit

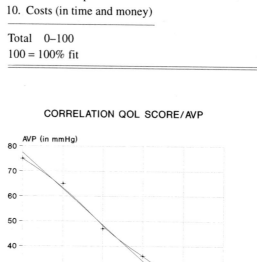

CORRELATION QOL SCORE/AVP

AVP (in mmHg)

Quality of Life Score

—⁺— mmHg Curve   —⁺— mmHg Trend

100 ▪ normality

Figure 1. Inverse correlation between the QOL score and the AVP measurement. This finding indicates that physiological and QOL assessments are in some way comparable.

venous incompetence (35%), deep venous incompetence without (30%) and with (5%) ulcerations and with mixed deep+superficial incompetence, it is possible to observe an inverse correlation between the QOL score and the AVP measurement (Figure 1). This confirms that physiological and QOL assessments are in some way comparable.

The correlation between years of venous diseases and QOL score shown in Figure 2 indicates a progressive deterioration of the QOL with the persistence of the venous disease and suggests that treatments useful for stopping or slowing down the progression of venous diseases may also act on the progressive deterioration of the QOL.

In a different series of 104 patients with symptomatic superficial and/or deep venous disease, it is possible to observe (Figure 3) that a decrease in AVP (after treatment) is inversely related to an increase in the QOL score (after treatment). These measurements of AVP and QOL were repeated 12 months after the appropriate treatment (surgery and/or sclerotherapy).

It is clear that there is a correlation, not always precise, between physiological parameters of venous insufficiency (i.e. AVP) and quality of

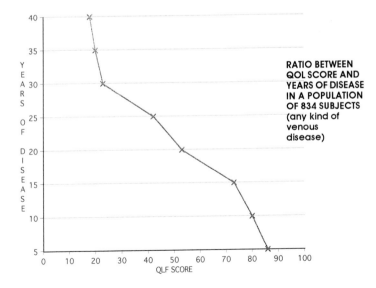

Figure 2. The correlation between years of venous diseases and QOL score shown. The graph indicates a progressive deterioration of the QOL with the persistence of the venous disease.

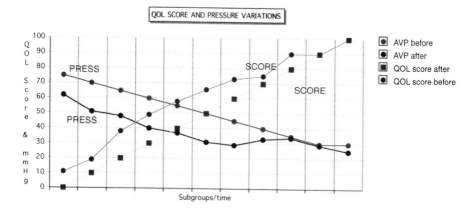

Figure 3. In a series of 104 patients with symptomatic superficial and/or deep venous disease it was possible to observe that a decrease in AVP (after treatment) was inversely related to an increase in the QOL score. The measurements of AVP and QOL were repeated 12 months after the appropriate treatment (surgery and/or sclerotherapy).

life. The future evaluation of treatments and management procedures of venous disorders must consider this new evaluation approach.

Finally, there is possibly an important correlation between diet and vascular diseases. Whilst in the past attention has been focused on the arterial side, there is now some evidence suggesting that diet may also be involved in the genesis of some venous disorders. If we observe (in a sample of 400 subjects) the consumption of some "accessory food elements" i.e. olive oil, berries and roots, and fibre content, we can observe a very interesting trend. There is an increase in the incidence of venous diseases (including haemorrhoids) and the consumption of these three elements. Whether they may have direct effects, particularly in the growth phase, or they are just a marker or expression of a different quality of life, it is difficult to say at the moment.

In particular, roots and berries, a very common "accessory" food in many rural areas — where they are directly collected from the ground — contain many vitamins, flavonoids (in the pigmented part of the plants) and other pharmacologically interesting compounds (including some alkaloids). They (Figure 4) appear to be connected with the evolution of venous diseases and their consumption appears to be inversely correlated with the occurrence of venous diseases.

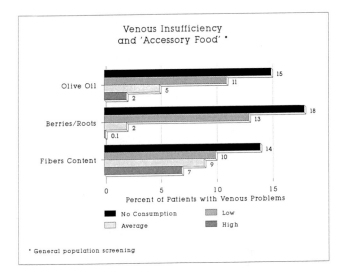

Figure 4. Olive oil, fibres and particularly roots and berries — a common "accessory" food in many rural areas — contain many vitamins, flavonoids (in the pigmented part of the plants) and other pharmacologically interesting compounds (including some alkaloids). They appear to be connected with the evolution of venous diseases and their consumption appears to be inversely correlated with the occurrence of venous diseases (including haemorroids).

Burkitt's observation that the content of fibres in the diet may be inversely proportional to the occurrence of some venous disorders may have followed this line of speculation. However, the inverse correlation of fibre intake and venous disease is less clear in our study.

In conclusion, venous disorders are common and tend to alter the quality of life of many otherwise healty subjects for a long period of time. New, noninvasive investigation methods useful for screening, the evaluation of the quality of life in subjects with venous diseases, and some new, interesting considerations (i.e. diet elements) are interesting options for the research in this field in the next few years. The preservation of a healthy venous system and preventing early and progressive deterioration is an important aim. It is now possible to avoid reaching the symptomatic stage by controlling most venous diseases in the subclinical phase. Whether this is possible at acceptable social costs will be the aim of our future clinical research.

The diffusion, through a simple but complete textbook, of our way of seeing, evaluating, preventing and treating most venous disorders will possibly be useful for promoting more attention to these common — often neglected — clinical problems before their human and social costs become too high for our communities.

CHAPTER 1

THE VENOUS SYSTEM

Venous Anatomy

Veins (particularly the veins of the lower limbs) can be classified into three groups:

(a) Superficial veins.
(b) Deep (muscular) veins which drain the gastrocnemius and soleus muscle of the calf; they are also generally considered within the deep venous system.
(c) Perforating or communicating veins.

Superficial veins

Superficial veins (Figures 1.1–1.3) in the leg are mainly the long and short saphenous vein systems. The term "saphenous" is probably a derivative of the Greek word *saphis*, which means "clearness", referring to the superficial course of the veins which makes them very evident. The long saphenous vein (LSV) is the longest vein of the body, its course originating from anterior to the medial malleolus, ascending along the medial part of the the leg and thigh to terminate in the common femoral vein at the groin. The LSV receives several tributaries. The most important are:

(1) The posterior arch vein (Leonardo's vein), which joins the LSV at the medial aspect of the knee. It is important because it is connected to the deep venous system by two or three constant ankle perforating veins (Cockett's perforators) (Figure 1.2).
(2) The anterior superficial tibial (or anterior saphenous) vein, which joins the long saphenous at the same level (or just below) as the posterior arch vein.

1

(3) In the thigh two long tributaries may be present, i.e. the antero-lateral (or anterior) and the postero-medial (or posterior) vein, which join the LSV near its termination. The postero-medial vein often connects with the upper part of the short saphenous vein (SSV) just before its entrance into the deep fascia. Common tributaries that join the long saphenous at the level of its junction with the deep system are the superficial circumflex iliac veins, the superficial inferior epigastric veins and the superficial external pudendal veins. There are often variations of anatomy at the junctions of the tributaries with the LSV.

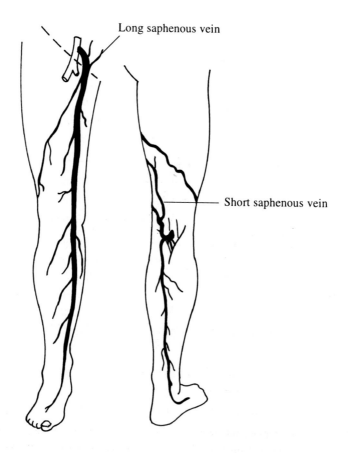

Long saphenous vein

Short saphenous vein

Figure 1.1. The long (internal) saphenous vein system (*left*) and the short (external) saphenous vein system (*right*).

greater long or int

The *lesser (short or external) saphenous vein (SSV)* begins at the outer border of the foot behind the lateral malleolus and ascends in the middle of the calf to the popliteal fossa, where it perforates the deep fascia to join the popliteal vein. The level of termination of the SSV is highly variable, with more than 30% terminating high up in the thigh. There is also considerable variation in the point where it perforates the fascia. It is, therefore, advisable to localise the junction with Duplex or venogram before sapheno-popliteal ligation.

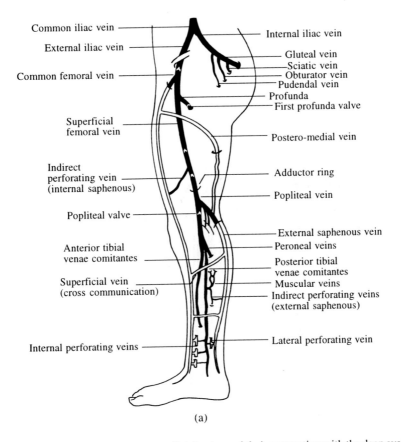

(a)

Figure 1.2. (a) The most important superficial veins and their connection with the deep system; (b) the most important connecting points between the deep and the superficial system; (c) the distal, below-knee superficial system (long saphenous vein); (d) the short, external saphenous system.

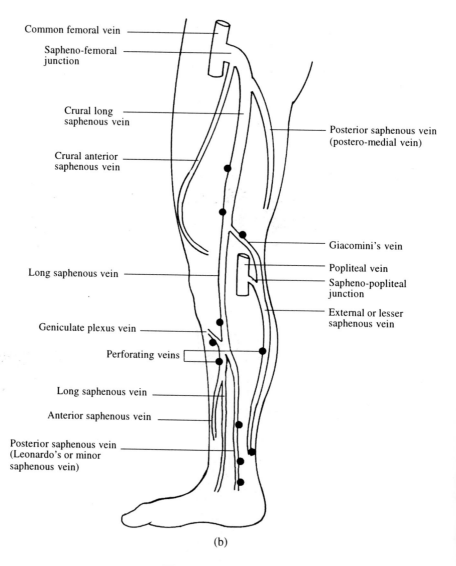

(b)

Figure 1.2 (*continued*)

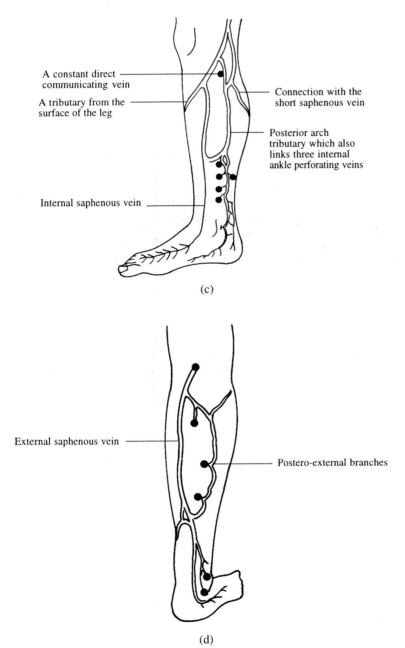

A constant direct communicating vein

A tributary from the surface of the leg

Internal saphenous vein

Connection with the short saphenous vein

Posterior arch tributary which also links three internal ankle perforating veins

(c)

External saphenous vein

Postero-external branches

(d)

Figure 1.2 (*continued*)

Deep veins

The deep veins of the lower limbs consist of three paired stems which run as venae comitantes along the corresponding arteries. They are the anterior tibial veins, the posterior tibial veins and the peroneal (fibular) veins. The posterior tibial veins receive the important medial ankle perforators from the posterior arch vein. The stem veins merge at the upper part of the calf to form the popliteal vein. The superficial femoral vein is the continuation of the popliteal vein after it has passed through the adductor canal. The deep femoral vein joins the superficial femoral vein 8–10 cm below the inguinal ligament to form the common femoral vein. The common femoral vein continues upwards, passes posteriorly to the inguinal ligament and becomes the external iliac vein. The superficial venous system joins the deep at the saphenofemoral junction and saphenopopliteal junctions. There are considerable variations in the anatomy of the deep veins. It has been suggested that the classical anatomical pattern is present in only 16% of limbs (Vasdekis).

The muscular veins drain mainly the gastrocnemious and soleus muscles. Their position at the center of the calf muscle pump mechanism gives them great importance in the normal function of the *venous pump*. The gastrocnemius veins drain the two heads of the gastrocnemius muscle and terminate by joining the popliteal vein at the level of the saphenopopliteal junction (or they may join the SSV). There are usually two veins, one emerging from the lateral head and one from the medial head of the gastrocnemius muscle. The medial one is frequently double. The variations of the anatomy and the communications of the veins with the other veins of the popliteal fossa can be demonstrated by colour duplex or venography, which may also show the presence or absence of valves in these veins. The termination of the gastrocnemius veins is, in approximately 30% of cases, in common with the short saphenous vein at the level of the saphenopopliteal junction. Distally the gastrocnemius communicates with the SSV through a mid-calf perforating vein at the site often called the *gastrocnemius point*. The other group of muscular veins drain the soleus muscle. They are large, sausage-shaped vessels usually without valves (soleal sinusoids). They join the posterior tibial and peroneal veins or the lower part of the popliteal vein.

Perforating or communicating veins

The two terms are synonymous. These veins perforate the fascia connecting the superficial with the deep venous system. They may be *direct*, i.e. those passing straight from the superficial vein to the main deep veins, or *indirect*, when the connection is via a muscle sinusoid. Anatomical dissections have indicated that more than 100 perforating veins may exist in one limb but very few are the important ones that may become incompetent and cause clinical problems. Incompetence of such calf perforating veins may be secondary to other sites of superficial incompetence and may revert to normal if these other sites are ligated. The main ones that connect the LSV with the deep veins are (in ascending order):

(1) *Cockett's perforating veins* are considered the most important perforating veins. They lie on a perpendicular line (Linton's line) behind the medial malleolus and connect the posterior arch veins with the posterior tibial veins. They are usually three in number (lower, middle and upper) and can be found at an almost constant average distance of 6, 13.5 and 18.5 cm respectively above the tip of the medial malleolus (indicated with a dot in Figure 1.2). In addition to these, another perforating vein may be present above the upper one (the *24 cm perforator*).

(2) *Boyd's perforating veins* are observed at the level of the tibial tuberosity, and connect the main trunk of the LSV with the posterior tibial veins, or sometimes with a branch of the gastrocnemius veins.

(3) *Dodd's perforating veins or thigh perforators* include a group of perforating veins connecting the LSV or an accessory LSV with the femoral vein. They may occur at any site on the medial aspect of the thigh, but the majority are found in the middle third of the thigh.

Another important group of perforating veins connect the SSV with the deep veins. They include:

(1) A constant perforating vein joining the SSV with the peroneal vein approximately at 5 cm above the os calcis (*Bassi's perforants*).

(2) The *soleus point*, a perforator connecting the soleus veins with the superficial veins of the calf.

(3) The *gastrocnemius point* (or *blow-out*) is an important perforating vein because of the aching symptoms it may produce in the presence of

incompetence. It connects the gastrocnemious vein with the superficial system (the SSV and its tributaries). This vein becomes incompetent secondary to insufficiency of the gastrocnemius vein.

Capillaries

The arteries gradually decrease in size to form the small arteries, the arterioles, and finally to end in the capillaries. The name *capillary* comes from the Latin *capillus*. The use of "capillary" to designate extremely small vessels, like a hair, has been attributed to Leonardo da Vinci in his 15th century writings. Capillaries are interposed between the smallest branches of the arteries and the commencing veins to constitute a network. They are present in all organs of the body with the exception of tendons. Their diameter differs in the various organs but the capillaries of the skin are the largest. The average size of capillaries in the body is 8 μm. Their network consists of capillaries in loops or elongated forms, depending upon the function of the organ. The wall of a capillary is formed by a layer of endothelial cells supported on its outside by a thin continuous basal lamina of collagen. Depending on the structure of the wall, capillaries are divided into the following categories:

(1) Continuous capillaries;
(2) Fenestrated capillaries;
(3) Sinusoid capillaries.

Continuous capillaries are present in muscles, nervous tissue and lungs. *Fenestrated and sinusoid capillaries* permit rapid exchange of substances and can be found in kidneys, cardiac muscle, liver and other organs where an increased filtration rate is necessary. The exchange of substances takes place through pores in the capillary membrane. It seems that there are two minute passageways serving this function:

(1) The intercellular cleft, which is a thin slit that lies between adjacent endothelial cells;
(2) The pinocytic channel, consisting of pinocytic vesicles that carry large molecules through the capillary membrane.

Venous Physiology

The venous system of the legs may be dynamically divided into four subsystems:

(1) The deep venous system;
(2) The superficial venous system;
(3) The perforating, communicating system;
(4) The microcirculation and the venular system.

Problems causing venous insufficiency may be localized in one or more than one of these systems. The deep venous system includes veins within the muscular compartments, beneath the deep fascia. It returns some 85% of the blood delivered to the leg. The superficial system (located in the subcutaneous tissue, superficially to the deep fascia) includes the greater and lesser saphenous vein systems with their tributaries. The perforating, communicating vein system includes veins perforating the fascia, connecting the deep to the superficial system. In normal perforating veins, valves direct flow from the superficial to the deep veins. Venous valves in the lower extremity are bicuspid, more numerous distally and less common proximally. The valves are not usually found in the iliac veins.

Venous pressure. In normal individuals on standing, the zero level of venous pressure is at the level of the right atrium. The hydrostatic pressure in a vein on the dorsum of the foot is equal to the distance from the right atrium to the foot — about 100 cm H_2O. In more distal veins the hydrostatic pressure is higher and the vein wall is proportionally thicker in consideration of the calibre of the vein. Muscular contractions continuously compressing the deep veins force blood toward the heart since the valves prevent retrograde flow. With muscular relaxation, the pressure in the deep venous systems decreases and the veins fill passively with blood. Efficient muscular action contributes to maintaining low levels of venous pressure.

In a normal limb, during walking, venous pressure decreases to about 30 mm H_2O (Figure 1.3) from a resting venous pressure of approximately 100–120 mm H_2O. The decrease in venous pressure is maintained until the end of the exercise, after which the intravenous pressure returns slowly to the pre-exercise level.

As a consequence of chronic venous disease with chronic venous hypertension, the increased venous pressure is transmitted to the venules and the microcirculation and the pathologic process affects the skin and subcutaneous tissues.

In chronic venous insufficiency the capillary network is altered. The increased exchange surface is due to elongation and dilatation of the capillaries which assume a glomerulus-like appearance with thickening of the capillary wall.

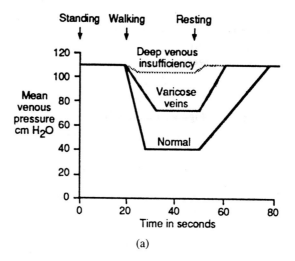

(a)

Figure 1.3. (a) Variations in venous pressure (in cm H_2O) with walking. The decrease in pressure in a normal venous system is shown in comparison with a system with varicose veins and deep (popliteal) venous incompetence. The degree of venous incompetence is mainly indicated by the refilling time at the end of the exercise test. Refilling is very fast if retrograde filling of the venous system occurs as a result of incompetence. The decrease in venous pressure is mainly due to outflow and it may be altered by obstruction. In severe deep obstruction and/ or incompetence, venous pressure may increase during exercise, leading to venous claudication. (b) The equivalent venous pressure curve (AVP) during and after exercise (in mmHg) is also shown. In the case of venous insufficiency the pressure decrease with exercise is less evident and the refilling time at the end of the exercise is very short (as the veins fill from above). A cuff excluding the superficial venous system will normalize the previous AVP curve, suggesting that the problem is only superficial and that the deep system is competent.

Ambulatory Venous Pressure and Refilling Time (R/T)
(patient with superficial venous incompetence)

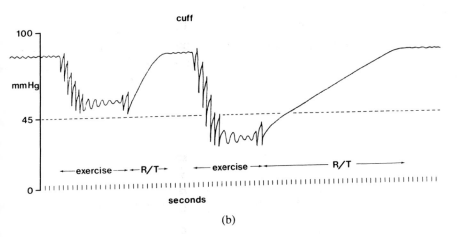

(b)

Figure 1.3 (*continued*)

CHAPTER 2

DIAGNOSTIC TESTS IN VENOUS INSUFFICIENCY

Noninvasive Testing

Chronic venous insufficiency (CVI) may be the result of outflow obstruction, reflux, or a combination of the two. The first objective of assessment is to detect whether obstruction or reflux is present. Second, the anatomic localization of the abnormality must be found, and finally the problem of quantification of the reflux or obstruction must be addressed. Where possible noninvasive tests are preferred. For the most part, these tests are widely available, simple, quick and cost-effective.

It should be noted that different tests may provide answers to different questions and that some are principally research tools.

In most clinical situations enough information can be obtained using a combination of only three techniques.

(1) Pocket Doppler;

(2) Colour duplex scanning;

(3) Air plethysmography (APG).

Tests for venous reflux. Venous reflux is the result of gravity drawing the venous blood stream distally. Therefore, reflux testing should be performed with the patient standing. Recent studies have determined that venous reflux detected in the supine position is frequently ended when the patient is standing, because valve closure occurs only after reflux exceeds a critical flow velocity.

When the patient is standing, it is important that muscular contractions be avoided. Therefore, the patient should be examined holding onto a frame or table. The leg to be examined should be relaxed with the knee slightly flexed, with the weight on the opposite leg. Studies have shown that during full knee extension, an occlusion of the popliteal vein occurs in 20% of healthy people. After the *clinical examination*, a *pocket Doppler* instrument is used. The pocket instruments are satisfactory for complementing the physical examination as a screening test for outpatients. The continuous wave instrument provides information about reflux at the sapheno-femoral and sapheno-popliteal junctions. The knee of the leg to be examined should be slightly flexed to relax the muscles and skin over the popliteal fossa. Manual calf compression produces cephalad flow and reflux may occur when the compression is released. Ending the reflux by compression of the superficial veins just below the probe suggests that reflux is confined to the superficial system. Failure to stop reflux by such a manoeuvre indicates that the reflux is in the deep system.

In experienced hands, a pocket Doppler is an important screening method which provides clear answers regarding the presence or absence of reflux at the sapheno-femoral and sapheno-popliteal junctions in most patients. Abnormal anatomy in the popliteal fossa is responsible for most of the errors (8%). For example, reflux in the gastrocnemius veins may be interpreted as reflux in the popliteal vein. Also, continuous wave Doppler is not accurate in localizing incompetent perforating veins.

Duplex and colour duplex scanning are more effective and faster that the examination with the pocket Doppler instrument. Duplex scanning provides information about reflux in specific veins. For example, the femoral, popliteal, deep calf veins and perforating veins can be individually tested. The use of colour has made duplex scanning faster and more accurate.

As in examination of a patient with the continuous wave instrument, the patient is examined standing. The non-weight-bearing lower extremity is evaluated and the sites to be studied are imaged with a 7.5 MHz (or low penetration) probe. The sapheno-femoral junction, the popliteal venous anatomy, the sapheno-popliteal junction and the perforating veins are visualized. Manual calf compression (or compression by a rapidly deflatable cuff) is used. The cuff inflation produces cephalad flow [Figure 2.1(a)], usually visualized in blue. Rapid release of the compression is essential to testing for reflux [Figure 2.1(b)] or to showing competence (absence reflux) or valve closure. Figure 2.2 shows the sapheno-popliteal junction and the veins in the popliteal fossa.

The Venous Clinic

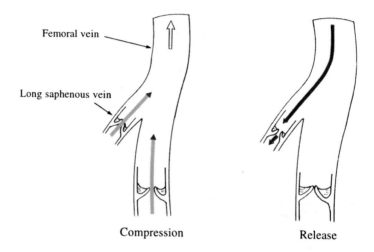

Femoral vein

Long saphenous vein

Compression   Release

Figure 2.1. Evaluation of the sapheno-femoral junction with colour duplex. Venous flow in the sapheno-femoral junction is shown during a manual compression-release manoeuvre of the thigh. Blue colour on calf compression indicates cephalad flow. Reflux is indicated by red colour on release of the compression.

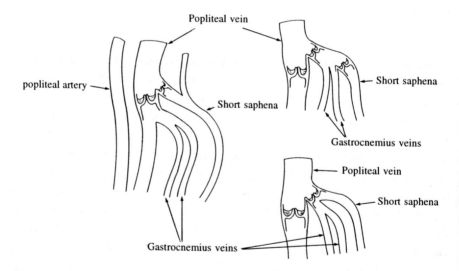

Popliteal vein

popliteal artery

Short saphena

Short saphena

Gastrocnemius veins

Popliteal vein

Short saphena

Gastrocnemius veins

Figure 2.2. The veins in the popliteal space. Three different but common anatomic variations of the veins in the popliteal fossa are shown. Duplex scanning reveals the anatomy and enables testing of each vein for reflux.

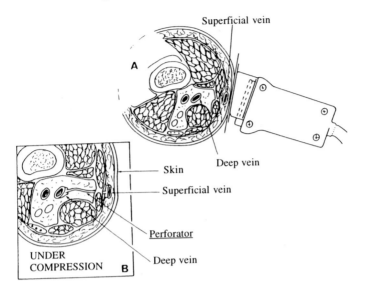

Figure 2.3. Transverse colour duplex of superficial and deep veins (A); by moving the probe up or down the limb with continuous visualization of the two veins, the presence and level of communicating veins are determined (B). The direction of flow with calf compression-release can then be tested. In incompetent perforating veins the flow visualization is easy, large and bidirectional.

In chronic venous insufficiency causing ulceration, the localization of perforating veins causing venous hypertension may be very important. In Figure 2.3 the localization of calf perforating veins and reflux in them is shown.

Colour duplex scanning is the most useful single test for assessment of venous pathology in the leg. Such an examination confirms the presence of reflux and its localization, morphology and function of deep veins and the extent and site of venous reflux, when present. Both localized and generalized reflux can be identified. Quantification of reflux in individual veins by duplex is possible, but the procedure is very time-consuming. Accurate and repro-ducible quantitative results are obtained easily for the whole leg using air plethysmography, which has become the test of choice for quantifying reflux.

Ambulatory venous pressure. Ambulatory venous pressure (AVP) measurement is regarded as a gold standard to which other examinations are compared. It is minimally invasive. Venous pressure is measured by inserting a needle in a vein on the dorsum of the foot with the patient standing (Figure 2.4). Pressures are recorded during a standard ten-tiptoe exercise test and AVP is defined as the lowest pressure reached during the exercise. AVP is a function of the calf muscle pump ejecting capacity, the magnitude of reflux and the outflow resistance. Therefore, it represents the net effect of all the abnormalities that affect venous haemodynamics. In normal limbs, the AVP is less than 30 mmHG and the refill time (RT) is greater than 18 sec. In normal limbs these values are due to filling of the veins from the arterial side. When venous reflux is present, the AVP is generally higher and the RT is shortened (Table 2.1). After AVP is obtained, the exercise test can be repeated with tourniquets (2.5 cm wide) applied at the ankle, below-knee or thigh positions. Tourniquets control reflux from the superficial veins, and if superficial reflux is present, the AVP and RT are normalized. In patients with deep venous incompetence, normalization does not occur.

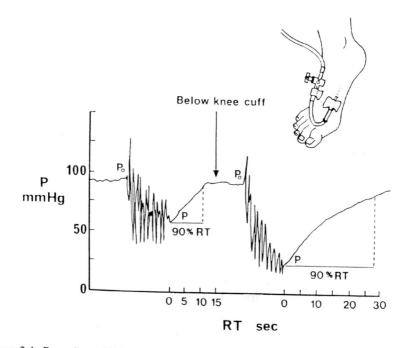

Figure 2.4. Recording of AVP during ten-tiptoe exercises with and without a below-knee cuff (2.5 cm wide) that occluded the superficial vein. Normalization of ambulatory venous pressure (P) and RT90 indicates that the deep veins are competent.

Table 2.1. Ambulatory venous pressure (AVP) and refilling time (RT).[*]

Type of limb	AVP (mmHg)		RT$_{90}$ (sec)	
	No ankle cuff	Ankle cuff	No ankle cuff	Ankle cuff
Normal	15–30	15–30	18–40	18–40
Primary varicose veins with competent perforating veins	25–40	15–30	10–18	18–35
Primary varicose veins with incompetent perforating veins	40–70	25–60[†]	5–15	8–30
Deep venous reflux (incompetent popliteal valves)	55–85	50–80	3–15	5–15
Popliteal reflux and proximal occlusion	60–110	60–120		
Popliteal occlusion and competent popliteal valves	25–60	10–60		

[*]Standard exercise: ten-tiptoe movements.
[†]In one third of these limbs, AVP remained more than 40 mmHg and RT$_{90}$ less than 15 sec despite the application of the ankle cuff.

Table 2.2. Incidence of ulceration in relation to ambulatory venous pressure (AVP) in 222 patients (251 limbs).

AVP (mmHg)	N	Incidence of ulceration
<30	34	0
30–40	44	11
41–50	51	22
51–60	45	38
61–70	34	59
71–80	28	68
81–90	10	60
>90	5	100

Table 2.1 indicates that AVP is higher than normal in the presence of popliteal reflux. For AVPs of 40–100 mmHg, there is a linear relationship to the incidence of skin ulceration. This is true regardless of the underlying pathology and whether the reflux is in the superficial or the deep system (Table 2.2).

Photoplethysmography (PPG) and light reflection rheography (LRR). In an attempt to obtain RT noninvasively, PPG and LRR tests were devised. In both of these techniques, a photodetector is applied to the skin of the foot or ankle (Figure 2.5). These methods determine whether venous incompetence is superficial or deep. Table 2.3 shows the PPG refilling times with and without an ankle cuff to occlude superficial veins in normal controls, patients with superficial reflux, and those with deep venous incompetence. Better reproducibility and better separation of groups can be obtained when the test is performed with the patient standing (as for AVP). It should be emphasized that both RT and RT_{90} (90% refilling time) obtained with PPG or LRR are poor measures of the severity of deep venous disease, as for a wide range of AVPs (i.e. between 40 and 100 mmHg), the RT_{90} is between 5 and 10 sec. Therefore a reduction in AVP from 100 to 60 mmHg, i.e. by valvuloplasty or valve substitution, may have a very limited effect on RT_{90}.

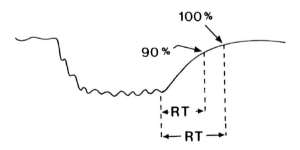

Figure 2.5. Measurement of RT or RT_{90} using photoplethysmography or light reflection rheography.

Table 2.3. Photoplethysmographic (PPG and LRR) refilling time (RT_{90}) with and without an ankle cuff to occlude superficial veins.

	Standing (sec)		Sitting (sec)	
	No cuff	Cuff	No cuff	Cuff
Normal	18–80*	18–80	26–100	26–100
SVI	5–18	18–50	2–25	18–50
DVI	3–12	6–18†	2–28	2–30

*$RT_{90} > 18$ sec without cuff identifies normal limbs.
†$RT_{90} < 18$ sec with cuff identifies limbs with deep venous incompetence.

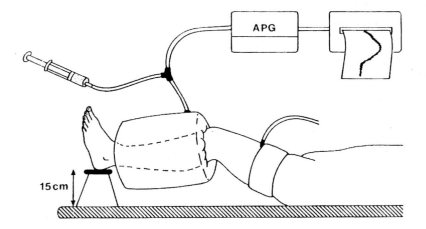

Figure 2.6. The APG (air plethysmograph). The 100 mL syringe included in the circuit is used for volume calibration.

Air plethysmography (APG) uses a calibrated air chamber applied to encompass the leg (Figure 2.6). It provides quantitative information about the various components of the calf muscle pump. These include:

• The rate of filling of the reservoir [venous filling index (VFI)] as a result of standing;

- The venous volume (VV), which is the amount of blood in the venous reservoir;
- The ejected volume (EV) and the ejection fraction (EF = EV/VV × 100) as a result of a single step;
- The residual volume (RV) and residual volume fraction (RVF = RV/VV × 100) as a result of ten-tiptoe movements.

The manoeuvres and methods of making these measurements from the recording are shown diagrammatically in Figure 2.7. Both the superficial system and the deep system can be evaluated. The presence of deep venous obstruction is also indicated [Figure 2.7(b)] by the venous outflow curve.

There is a high reproducibility of measurements expressed as ratios: VFI, EF and RVF (coefficient of variation less than 10%) (Table 2.4). VFI is a measurement of reflux and is expressed in ml per second. Volume measurements are in absolute units (millilitres). The median and 90% range of the various measurements in different groups of patients are shown in Figure 2.8 and in Table 2.4.

The linear correlation that exists between the RVF and the AVP (Figure 2.9) indicates that an estimate of the AVP can be obtained noninvasively from the RVF. The incidence of cutaneous ulceration increases with an increase in the amount of reflux (VFI) and a decrease in the efficiency of the calf muscle pump ejection (EF). Thus, the RFV provides information on the overall effect of all the venous abnormalities. In addition, the abnormalities are dissected out and measured in terms of the EF (ejection) and the VFI (reflux) components.

Tests for outflow obstruction. Ascending venography remains the standard method of delineating persistent venous obstruction and demonstrating its anatomy. There are several noninvasive tests that determine the presence and quantify the degree of outflow obstruction. The simple continuous wave Doppler measurement can be used as a screening device in outpatients. A history of deep venous thrombosis or persistent leg and ankle swelling suggests the need for such an examination. Although not in general worldwide use, the best test for evaluating obstruction is the *arm–foot pressure differential developed by Raju, which is an invasive test.* Other noninvasive tests are based on the measurements of venous outflow by various techniques using different instrumentation. These methods include the strain gauge, impedance plethysmography and APG, which has become the method of choice. However, the other methods are in more general and worldwide use.

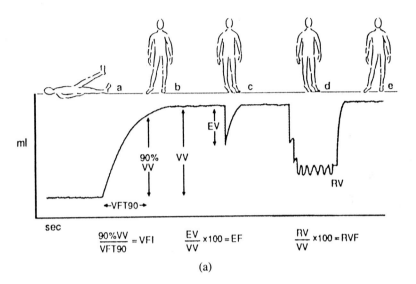

$$\frac{90\%\,VV}{VFT90} = VFI \qquad \frac{EV}{VV} \times 100 = EF \qquad \frac{RV}{VV} \times 100 = RVF$$

(a)

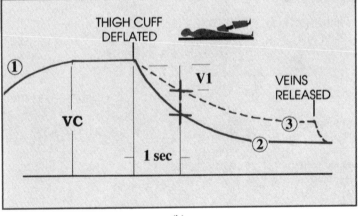

(b)

Figure 2.7. (a) The manoeuvres and methods of deriving the APG measurements. Both the superficial system and the deep system can be evaluated. The presence of deep venous obstruction is indicated (b) by the venous outflow curve. 1 = inflow curve; 2 = outflow (normal); 3 = outflow decreased by obstruction; VC = venous capacitance.

Table 2.4. Air plethysmography.

	Units	Coefficient of variation	Normal limbs	Primary VV's	DVD
Direct measurements					
Functional venous volume (VV) (increase in leg volume on standing)	mL	10.8–12.5	100–150	100–350	70–320
Venous filling time (VFT90) (time taken to reach 90% of VV)	sec	8.0–11.5	70–170	5–70	5–20
Ejected volume (EJ) (decrease in leg volume as a result of one tiptoe)	mL	6.7–9.4	60–150	50–180	8–140
Residual volume (RV) (volume of blood left in veins after ten tiptoes)	mL	6.2–12	2–45	50–150	60–200
Derived measurements					
Venous filling index (VFI) (average filling rate: 90% VF/VFT90)	mL/sec	5.3–8	0.5–1.7	2–25	7–30
Ejection fraction (EF = EV/VV × 100)	%	2.9–9.5	60–90	25–70	20–50
Residual volume fraction (RVF = RV/VV × 100)	%	4.3–8.2	2–35	25–80	30–100

VV's = Varicose veins
DVD = Deep venous disease

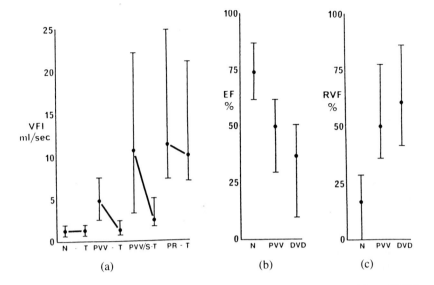

(a)   (b)   (c)

Figure 2.8. (a) VFI in normal controls, limbs with primary varicose veins without (PVV) and with skin changes (PVV/S), and limbs with popliteal reflux (PR). The results are presented as median and 90% range without and with a 2.5 cm tourniquet (T) at the knee that occluded the superficial veins. The application of this tourniquet can differentiate between reflux in the superficial and deep veins. (b) Ejection fraction (EF) in normal controls, limbs with primary varicose veins (PVV) and deep venous disease (DVD) (median and 90% range). (c) Residual volume fraction (RVF) in the same group of patients.

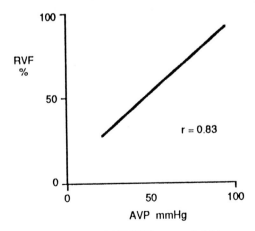

Figure 2.9. Correlation between AVP and RVF (SVI = superficial incompetence; DVD = deep venous disease).

Ultrasound methods

Continuous wave (CW) Doppler and duplex scanning. CW Doppler is only a screening procedure and cannot be considered diagnostic for outflow obstruction. The patient is examined with the legs horizontal and the knees slightly flexed. The trunk should be at 45° and the ultrasound probe is held over the femoral vein. Flow velocity is normally phasic with respiration. If this is found, it indicates a normal iliocaval segment. Absence of phasic flow or the finding of flow that is continuous and not affected by respiration suggests obstruction. If flow is diminished or stopped by compression of the contralateral groin or suprapubic area, the presence of obstruction and collateral circulation is established. Augmentation of the velocity in the common femoral vein by calf compression indicates absence of popliteal and femoral venous obstruction. This manoeuvre can be repeated with occlusion of the long saphenous vein at the knee by external pressure. This double-checks the patency of the popliteal vein. Augmentation of the velocity in the popliteal vein produced by digital compression of each venous compartment in the leg suggests patent axial deep calf vein flow.

B-mode ultrasound, duplex and colour duplex imaging detect with great accuracy veins containing organized thrombus that are not compressible by probe pressure. Such visualization of the deep veins may even reveal irregular vein walls with abnormal echo patterns and partially recanalized lumens. Also, the density (echogenicity) of the thrombus may be an indication of its age as fresh clot is very echolucent (same density and appearance of blood) and old clots (3–4 weeks and more) are echogenic.

Arm–foot pressure differential (Raju). The arm–foot pressure differential measurement is considered to be the gold standard method of quantitating outflow obstruction. This technique consists in recording the venous pressure in the veins of the foot and hand simultaneously after venous cannulation. The measurements are made with the patient supine and are repeated after inducing reactive hyperaemia in the leg. In normal limbs, the arm–foot pressure differential is less than 5 mmHg, with a rise of 1–6 mmHg (i.e. 5 may rise by 1–6 mmHg, to become 6–11 mmHg) during reactive hyperaemia. Patients with venographically proven evidence of obstruction have been classified into four grades according to the criteria shown in Table 2.5.

Table 2.5. Arm–foot differential (P mmHg) in limbs with outflow obstruction.

Grade	Pressure at rest	Pressure increment during hyperaemia
I: Fully compensated	<5	<6
II: Partially compensated	<5	<6
III: Partially decompensated	>5	>6 (often 10–15)
IV: Fully decompensated	>>>5 (often 15–20)	No further increase

Outflow measurements. The degree of venous obstruction can be assessed from outflow measurements using mercury strain gauge or air plethysmography. In both techniques, a proximal thigh cuff is inflated with the patient supine and the limb elevated 10° with external rotation and 10° knee flexion. The veins are allowed to fill for at least 2 min and the cuff is suddenly deflated. Measurements are made from the outflow curves. Maximum venous outflow, 1 sec outflow, and 3 sec outflow fractions are all valid measurements used and advocated by different authors. The outflow fraction is expressed as $OF = V_1/VV \times 100$ (20).

Table 2.6 shows the range of values for limbs with normal veins, moderate and also severe obstruction for strain gauge plethysmography (MVO) and air plethysmography (OF). The correlation between the outflow fraction using air plethysmography and arm–foot pressure differentials is good ($r > 0.7$).

Table 2.6. Maximum venous outflow (MVO).

Obstruction	Normal	Moderate	Severe
MVO strain gauge (1sec) (mL/100 mL/min)	45	45–30	30
1 sec outflow fraction (OF) Air plethysmography (% of VV)	38	38–30	30

VV = Venous volume

Outflow resistance can be calculated from the APG and direct venous pressure outflow curves obtained simultaneously (Figure 2.10).

Outflow (Q) can be calculated from the tangent at any point on the volume outflow curve. Resistance ($R = P/Q$) is calculated by dividing the corresponding pressure (P) by the flow (Q). This can be done for a series of points on the outflow curves. By plotting the resistance against pressure it has been shown that the relation between these is not linear. At low pressures when the veins are collapsed, the resistance is high. The resistance decreases at higher pressures when the veins, and presumably the veins of the collateral circulation, are distended.

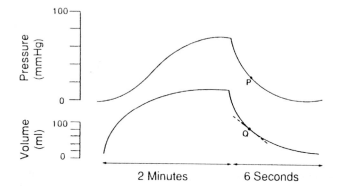

Figure 2.10. Pressure and volume inflow and outflow curves obtained simultaneously using an APG and cannulation of a vein on the dorsum of the foot.

Figure 2.11 demonstrates the relationship between the resistance and the four grades of arm–foot pressure differential described by Raju.

In conclusion, it is possible to detect noninvasively or minimally invasively the presence or absence of reflux or obstruction in venous circulation, the anatomic site and to obtain quantitative measurements of the severity of both. Acceptable information can be obtained using the pocket Doppler as a screening method, duplex and colour duplex scanning for morphology and localization and APG or AVP for quantification of reflux and/or obstruction.

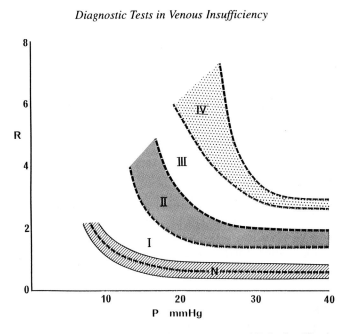

Figure 2.11. Relationship between outflow resistance curves and Raju classification of outflow obstruction (Grades I–IV) (N: normal limbs).

Invasive Tests

For patients who would be candidates for reconstructive surgery, further and more precise knowledge of morphology and function is necessary after noninvasive testing. It is critical to differentiate between venous obstruction and reflux and find out whether the reflux is due to primary valve incompetence with reparable deep valves or post-thrombotic with destroyed valves. In obstruction we need to assess pathways for various bypasses in the ilac or (rarely) the femoral veins. In iliac obstruction, ascending and descending phlebography combined with femoral venous pressure measurements are the invasive methods of choice.

Ascending phlebography is important in candidates for deep reconstruction. Ascending phlebography is also useful in patients with chronic venous insufficiency, mapping the patient's veins in the extremities and identifying the incompetent perforating veins in the calf. It will also identify obstructed venous segments in the calf, thigh and pelvis and most of the recanalized post-thrombotic segments. Further, ascending phlebography will provide a map of patent veins in the extremity. It is carried out by injecting contrast into a vein on the dorsum of the foot. The presence of an ankle touniquet directs the contrast into the deep veins. Good visualisation of the deep veins up to the vena cava can be obtained.

Descending phlebography is necessary for planning deep vein valve reconstruction or valve substitution procedures and is the only reliable means of differentiating primary valve incompetence (PVI) from secondary, post-thrombotic valve incompetence (SVI) as a cause of deep vein reflux in the proximal thigh. It is performed by the introduction of a cannula through a brachial, femoral or popliteal venous puncture and injection of contrast in the upright position using a tilting table. Individual study of the long saphenous vein, superficial femoral vein and profunda femoral vein is done to identify the presence of valves and their state of competence with and without Valsalva. When reflux occurs through a proximal valve the contrast is followed distally in that segment until it dissipates. The descending phlebogram is classified by considering the distal extent of reflux. When reflux is limited to the thigh veins the patient is not usually considered to be a candidate for deep vein valve surgery. When reflux passes through the popliteal vein and into the calf, surgical correction may be deemed appropriate. Because the descending phlebogram is a dynamic study, it is preferable to record a videotape of the study for future analysis. Bilateral femoral pressure measurements should be performed utilizing the cannulas, in the supine, resting position and during dorsovolar flexion. The most important indicators of functional obstruction of the iliac veins are pressure elevation after exercise, pressure difference after exercise and a slow pressure normalization time after exercise.

CHAPTER 3

SUPERFICIAL VENOUS INSUFFICIENCY AND VARICOSE VEINS

Diagnosis

- Dilated, tortuous superficial veins with irregular dilatations.
- Subjective symptoms are usually mild (fatigue, aching and moderate swelling, particularly in the evening) or absent. Signs and symptoms are usually partially relieved by leg elevation and disappear in the morning after a night's rest.
- Chronic varicosities may be associated with skin pigmentation and even ulceration. Severe signs and symptoms (i.e. distal chronic oedema) may be associated with secondary varicose veins.

Introduction and General Considerations

Varicose veins are dilated, elongated and tortuous veins in the subcutaneous tissue. They are incompetent as blood flow is not prevalently monodirectional–centripetal as in normal veins but mainly bidirectional–centrifugal. Varicosities are common in the lower extremities, but they also occur in other anatomic areas, i.e. the spermatic cord (varicocele), oesophagus (oesophageal varices) and anorectum (haemorrhoids). Some 10–20% of the world's population may have varicose veins in the legs. The prevalence varies according to the characteristics of the population as more primitive populations living an active life and feeding on a diet rich in fibre appear to have a low prevalence of varicose veins. On the contrary, the increased incidence of varicose veins and haemorroids correlates well with the low roughage diet consumed in most developed countries. Also, varicose veins are more frequent in patients with diverticular disease of the colon. They are probably more common in women. Other factors associated with an increased incidence of varicose veins appear to be pregnancy, constricting clothing, prolonged standing, obesity, and chronic treatment with oestrogens (the first generation of oral contraceptives).

Varicose veins are generally divided into *two classes: primary and secondary*. *Primary or simple varicose veins* are usually associated with a normal deep venous system while *secondary varicose veins* are considered to be a complication of deep venous disease usually associated with chronic venous obstruction (thrombosis, compression or obstruction or arteriovenous fistula).

Differentiating between superficial and/or deep incompetence and simple varicose veins is not easy. The definition of varicose veins is clinical. More correctly, the patients are considered to have (on the basis of dynamic, noninvasive tests) incompetence of the deep and/or superficial system. Therefore varicose veins are considered to be an important but not exclusive sign of venous incompetence.

The causes of primary varicose veins are still unknown. Two major hypotheses, both unsatisfactory, have been developed. They overlap in most cases.

The valvular incompetence hypothesis. Valvular incompetence is the most important observation in superficial vein (particularly saphenous vein) varicosity. This factor appears to be the most important in determining the clinical course and progression of varicose veins. The fundamental abnormality is progressive, sequential incompetence of the valvular rings in the main saphenous trunks and in the communicating veins. The proximal incompetent valves produce continuous levels of high venous pressure on the more distal valve, causing in time segmental dilatation of that venous segment and of the more distal valvular ring which constitutes the distal end of that segment.

The weak wall hypothesis. This hypothesis suggests an inherited weakness of the vein wall, producing progressive venous dilatation even at normal venous pressure, with secondary failure of competence of the dilated valvular rings. In approximately 50% of patients there is a family history suggesting an inherited defect and simple varicose veins often first appear in teenage or early adult life.

Secondary varicosities usually develop after damage and chronic obstruction to the deep venous systems. After deep venous thrombosis the recanalization of the thrombosed veins may destroy the valvular cusps, leaving the venous segment incompetent. The loss of competence causes continuous venous reflux, leading to stretching and elevated pressure on the superficial veins. These veins have a weak external support from the subcutaneous tissue as they are superficial to the deep fascia of the leg. Following chronic deep obstruction, secondary varicosities progressively develop as a consequence of the increased venous pressure directly transmitted from the deep to the superficial venous system by the incompetent veins (including the perforating veins). Severe deep obstruction of a major venous segment — i.e. inferior vena cava, iliac and femoral veins — often results in diffuse secondary varicosities.

Suprapubic varicosities often represent residual collateral veins that develop after iliofemoral thrombosis with severe obstruction.

In some subjects *arteriovenous fistulas* may be the cause of regional varicose veins. This is indicated (using Doppler) by the presence of a continuous, high velocity venous flow (in normal veins the venous flow is phasic with respiration).

The *Klippel–Trenaunay syndrome* is a form of congenital arteriovenous malformation which may be associated with varicose veins of the lower extremities and absence or abnormal development of the deep veins.

Diagnosis

Diffuse, severe varicosity and skin complications may be associated with absence of subjective symptoms, while some patients may have symptoms even with small varicosities. Why this should be so is not understood. Frequently reported symptoms are leg aching and heaviness, cramps, and itching associated with swelling. Patients often complain only of the cosmetic aspects of the varicosities. Symptoms often occur after prolonged standing, are more severe in the evening and are partially or completely relieved by leg elevation, night rest or elastic compression (i.e. stockings).

The swelling associated with primary varicose veins is usually mild, localized at the ankle and foot, and disappears after leg elevation overnight.

In women signs and symptoms may be more significant in the few days just prior to menses.

Eczema, skin dryness and scaling dermatitis associated with pruritus are often observed over large varicose veins, especially distal (ankle and foot).

The symptoms of uncomplicated primary varicose veins are usually mild and most patients are referred only for cosmetic reasons. Varicose veins may be painful but severe pain or disability is rarely or never associated with primary varicose veins. Often these symptoms are associated with other problems (i.e. muscular, articular, neurological, obesity) and are not caused by the varicose veins. It is important to make clear to the patient that these symptoms will not disappear even after correct treatment of the varicose veins. Secondary varicose veins due to chronic deep venous insufficiency are often associated with some degree of obstruction and cause more severe symptoms. If chronic venous disease is not treated or controlled it may progress to venous ulceration in many patients. It is also important to consider that while most varicose ulcers are labelled as post-thrombotic, many ulcers (some 30–45%) may be simply due to chronic venous hypertension caused by pure superficial incompetence.

The signs and symptoms associated with *venous hypertensive microangiopathy* and skin complications are caused by the degree of chronic venous hypertension. A high level of venous hypertension may be caused even by simple, large varicose veins, which may lead to lipodermatosclerosis and ulceration as well as severe deep incompetence. Important haemorrhage from venous ulceration and perforators may occur spontaneously or following even minor trauma.

A general physical examination may reveal predisposing causes of varicosities or conditions (i.e. obesity). Inspection of legs in the standing position will indicate the localization of the most important varicose veins. In the case of oedema or obesity, veins may be difficult to observe but palpation and percussion along the course of the greater saphenous vein (Schwartz test) may be a useful diagnostic test.

It is good clinical practice to record the position of the varicose veins, and photographs of the veins before surgery may be very useful, especially for unusual vein patterns and for medico-legal documentation.

Mild pitting ankle oedema and slight pigmentation of the skin usually indicate a moderate, long-lasting venous hypertension and the need for treatment.

The *Brodie–Trendelenburg test* is used to test the competence of the perforating veins and those in the greater saphenous system. With the patient supine, the leg is elevated to drain blood from the superficial veins. The saphenous vein is then occluded with compression in the thigh and the patient stands up. After observing the varices for 30 sec the compression is removed. In normal limbs gradual filling of the superficial veins occurs from below on standing. When the tourniquet is removed the filling is very gradual. In the case of incompetence the veins fill rapidly through the incompetent perforators directly from the deep system. The location of the incompetent perforator veins can be determined by placing multiple tourniquets around the leg and thigh and observing which venous segments fill.

Competence of the sapheno-femoral junction is determined by removing the tourniquet around the proximal thigh. In the case of incompetence the reflux rapidly fills the greater saphenous system. The long saphenous system should be occluded when similarly testing the short saphenous vein by occluding it in the popliteal fossa. Palpation along and close to the the superficial varices is useful in identifying incompetent perforating veins (usually associated with palpable depressions in the fascia). Perforating veins are frequently seen in the lower leg just posterior to the tibia. The validity of the clinical examination of varicose veins is determined by the experience of the examiner. Noninvasive investigations (particularly screening with the simple continuous wave pocket Doppler) are very useful for ruling out major deep venous problems and for defining the major points of incompetence which need treatment. With a hand-held Doppler the presence or absence of incompetence of the sapheno-femoral junction and the junction between the short saphenous and popliteal veins can be quickly demonstrated in the venous clinic. The absence of reflux on a compression-release manoeuvre will almost always rule out venous incompetence. The presence of reflux indicates a more careful and detailed evaluation with colour duplex. It is good practice to have a pocket Doppler available when seeing patients with varicose veins, as this simple examination will speed up the investigation process and avoid a number of unnecessary duplex investigations.

Differential diagnosis. Lipodermatosclerosis, hyperpigmentation with skin induration and venous ulceration are more often associated with chronic deep venous insufficiency and secondary varicosity than with primary varicose veins. Rarely, a thrill or bruit may indicate the presence a large arteriovenous fistula. These signs are usually absent in the case of small arterio-venous communications. Venous dilatations appearing suddenly or self-aggravating in a short period of time may be associated with problems causing extrinsic venous compression. These should particularly be considered in the inguinal and retroperitoneal areas and evaluated with abdominal ultrasound and CT or MRI scans when needed. Venous dilatation without real varicosity in one limb may be an indication of compression of the venous system (i.e. compression by a tumour by the right iliac artery crossing the left iliac vein).

Unilateral or bilateral swelling and oedema of the limbs may also be due to lymphatic problems and other clinical problems.

Complications

Acute complications of varicose veins are haemorrage and thrombosis. When the skin, especially in perimalleolar areas, becomes atrophic, the varices become very superficial and may bleed with even minor trauma. This may cause a large haemorrhage, which can be controlled by local compression and leg elevation. The sudden incompressibility of dilated veins (usually associated with local pain) is a sign that a varicose vein has thrombosed, causing thrombophlebitis.

Chronic complications are due to venous stasis causing chronic venous hypertension. Skin induration and hyperpigmentation (from the accumulation of haemosiderin) may finally lead to ulceration. Dermatitis, eczema and skin irritation are often associated with itching, and scratching lesions may be observed. The affected skin is more susceptible to cellulitis and local infections.

Treatment of Varicose Veins

The aims of the treatment of varicose veins are:

(1) To prevent stasis and its complications;

(2) To relieve signs and symptoms;

(3) To improve the appearance of the leg.

Most patients (particularly young women) ask for treatment mainly for cosmetic reasons rather than for real signs/symptoms, and this should be borne in mind when deciding on treatment strategy. The type of therapy to be used is also determined by the severity of the venous insufficiency. Some 30% of patients with simple varicosities do not require any therapy. Follow-up and advice is all that is needed.

Three different types of therapy are commonly used (most often in combination) to treat and control varicose veins:

(1) Physical measures (i.e. elastic compression);

(2) Surgery;

(3) Sclerotherapy.

In the treatment of varicose veins the following rules must be considered:

Rule 1. Venous insufficiency (of which varicose veins are a demonstration) is a chronic problem which is present during the entire patient's life. Therefore very often it is not possible to treat the problem with one single, isolated intervention. Patients are better treated with repeated, planned therapeutic interventions.

Rule 2. It is more realistic to consider that the chronic evolution of venous insufficiency can be controlled rather than definitely treated with either nonoperative management or surgery and/or compression sclerotherapy.

Rule 3. The three main treatment options must be well understood and logically applied in different phases of the disease and of the life of the patient.

Rule 4. Treatments must always be based on careful understanding of the problem based on the definition and localization of the dynamic alterations (incompetence and/or obstruction).

Rule 5. Noninvasive investigations are the basis of a correct treatment and treatment planning.

Rule 6. The treatment of varicose veins must always be planned bearing in mind that this problem is not a very dangerous condition for the patient. Therefore the incidence of complications and unsatisfactory results should be kept to a minimum and the cost of treatment should always be considered.

Physical measures aim to reduce stasis, improving venous return, and decrease the average venous pressure by shifting blood from the varicose superficial system to the deep veins. Walking and regular physical exercise is useful while prolonged standing and sitting should be avoided. Leg elevation whenever possible reduces venous pressure, and elastic stockings compress the superficial venous system reducing reflux and venous pooling from the deep to the superficial veins. Reflux through the incompetent perforators is also reduced by effective elastic compression. Below-knee stockings are very effective, as the highest venous pressure and the most important varicosities are localized below the knee. *Stockings (and bandages)* are not very effective in compressing thigh varicosities and perforators. Compression with elastic stockings is very helpful in controlling and preventing oedema and its consequences, also improving the ejection power of the calf muscle pump. Elastic bandages can be used for compression in the most severe cases but must be carefully applied by specialized staff to avoid a tourniquet effect. Exercise, leg elevation and stockings are effective in many patients with simple varicose veins. Relief of signs (particularly oedema) and subjective symptoms is generally rapidly obtained in the less severe forms of venous insufficiency. Even in patients with more severe chronic venous hypertension — due to superficial incompetence — physical measures are not only palliative but may constitute a very effective form of treatment when surgery or sclerotherapy is not possible, and/or patients refuse more aggressive forms of treatment.

Surgical treatment. Surgical treatment of varicose veins is indicated in the case of (a) important symptoms and signs; (b) very large varicosities which may thrombose, causing superficial thrombophlebitis; (c) complications and/or high risk of complications (i.e. history of superficial thrombophlebitis or haemorrhage from ruptured varices); (d) skin pigmentation, lipodermatosclerosis and/or ulcerations from chronic venous hypertension (often associated with deep venous incompetence); (e) cosmetic reasons.

Surgery for varicose veins aims to remove or ligate all, or the most important, varices and incompetent perforators. In the case of secondary varicosities associated with deep venous incompetence, the surgical removal of the incompetent superficial veins must always be associated with chronic physical treatment and whenever possible with deep venous correction or reconstruction. *Stripping* is a debatable but widely used procedure. Avoiding stripping may preserve a long saphenous vein which may later be used for a graft (peripheral vascular or coronary). However, a varicose saphenous vein is very seldom used for a graft, in which case there is little point in its preservation. In addition thigh perforators are usually disrupted by stripping resulting in a lessening of recurrence. It is therefore correct to use stripping when the whole long saphenous vein is varicose, usually from the groin to just below the knee. Stripping is sometimes performed down to the ankle but this may increase the incidence of damage to the saphenous nerve. All incompetent varicosities and perforating veins must be identified before surgery, with the patient standing. The varices are marked preoperatively (colour duplex can be helpful particularly in identifying perforators). Surgery may be performed under general or regional anaesthesia. It includes careful ligation of the greater saphenous vein and its tributaries at the sapheno-femoral junction, close to the femoral vein (Figure 3.1). If the vein is to be stripped this is then performed (Figure 3.2). Some visible varicosities are tributaries of the main trunk and therefore they are removed or interrupted by stripping. The remaining varicose veins and perforators are removed or ligated through separate multiple small skin incisions. The use of special hooks enables very small incisions to be made enhancing the cosmetic result. As an alternative, to avoid excessive skin incisions, smaller remaining varicosities can be

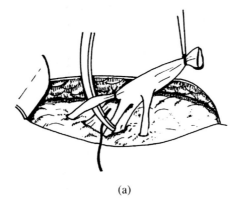

(a)

Figure 3.1. Ligation and section of the sapheno-femoral junction. The vein is isolated, ligated and sectioned (a,b). The collateral veins close to the junction are carefully isolated, ligated and cut (c). Finally, the vein is ligated (with a transfixing stitch) close to the femoral vein (d).

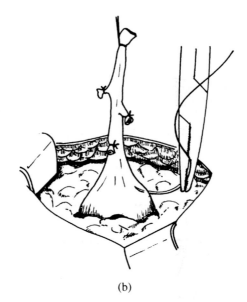

(b)

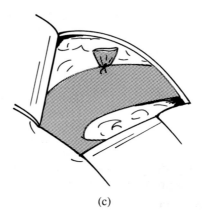

(c)

Figure 3.1 (*continued*)

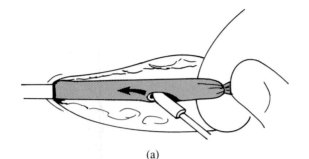

(a)

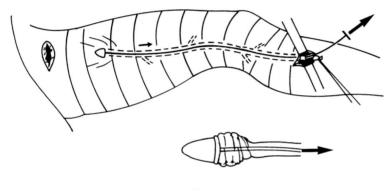

(b)

Figure 3.2. Introduction of the vein stripper into the distal long saphenous vein (a) at the ankle and stripping (b).

obliterated, after 1–3 weeks, by sclerotherapy. It is believed that once the main venous (high venous pressure) segments have been ligated or removed, most of the smaller (low venous pressure) tributaries tend to thrombose or disappear.

Subfascial ligation of the incompetent perforating veins obliterates the communication between the superficial and the deep system, further decreasing venous pressure and reducing the possibilities of recanalization of superficial venous branches. These careful steps are needed as stripping only does not remove many important venous segments and their communication with the most common perforators. When the incompetence is mainly localized to a segment of the long saphenous vein, limited stripping (associated with ligation of other incompetent venous sites) can be used (Figure 3.3). Limited stripping procedures are less traumatic, recovery is much faster and the method is suitable for use as an out-patient procedure. Additionally, limited stripping preserves the segments of veins which are not varicose. *Incompetence of the lesser saphenous systems* (Figure 3.4) is treated through an incision at the popliteal fold, just below the popliteal fossa and distally, behind the lateral malleolus (when stripping is required). Simple ligation of the vein at its junction with the popliteal vein is often effective in reducing or stopping varicosities in this territory. After a few weeks sclerotherapy of residual veins is very effective in this area.

As an alternative, stripping or multiple ligations of the incompetent veins (after ligating the sapheno-popliteal junction) are effective. Stripping of the lesser saphenous vein may be more difficult than stripping of the long saphenous vein and the occurrence of nerve damage may be higher. Recurrences are sometimes observed, as variations of the anatomy in this area are numerous. The sapheno-popliteal junction may be more proximal than expected. Ultrasound (colour duplex scanning) and in some instances (i.e. when surgery for recurrence is planned) intraoperative venography maybe very useful. These methods will correctly identify the branches present

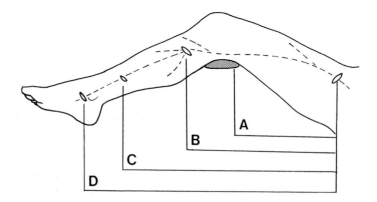

Figure 3.3. Different types of stripping are possible when varicosity is localized to a venous segment only. Short, selective stripping is less traumatic and patients usually do not need hospitalization.

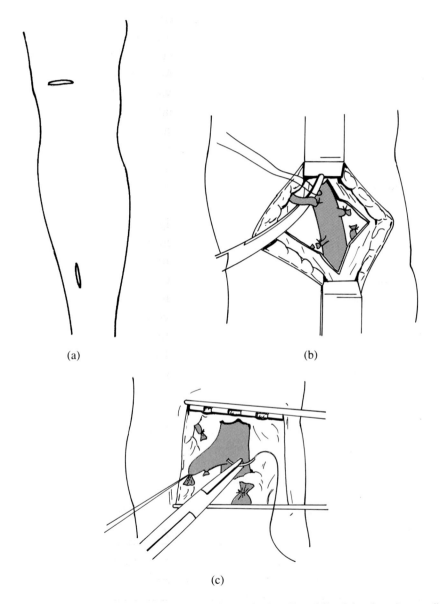

(a)

(b)

(c)

Figure 3.4. Position of the leg for ligation (1) or stripping (2 and 3) of the short (external) saphenous vein (a). Ligation of collateral veins (b) and of the sapheno-popliteal junction (c). *Note:* The size of incisions in the figure is larger than the real size for clarity.

in the popliteal area differentiating the popliteal vein and the gastrocnemius veins from the lesser saphenous vein and identifying its confluence into the deep system, which is quite variable. After stripping or ligation of the main incompetent venous segments, the smaller varices may be treated with transfixion (Figure 3.5). A small cotton swab is placed between the suture and the skin to avoid skin damage. The suture is removed after 3–5 days (depending on the size of the vein).

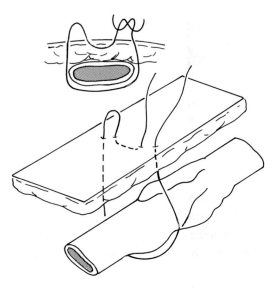

Figure 3.5. Transcutanous ligation (transfixion) of a small, residual varicosity after ligation and/or stripping of the larger varicose veins.

Injection sclerotherapy is also possible to obliterate collateral veins (Figure 3.6) after ligation of the larger varices. Finally, the most important perforating veins, identified before surgery, are ligated as shown in Figure 3.7. After surgery elastic bandages or, better still, graduated compression stockings are generally used for a few days (depending on the extension of stripping and mainly to avoid haematomas in the postoperative hours). Thigh length compression stockings or bandages are used for the following 2–4 weeks.

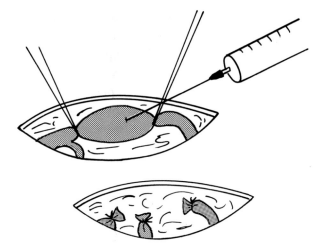

Figure 3.6. Intraoperative, retrograde sclerosing injection of a varicose collateral vein after ligation of the larger varicose trunks.

Physical measures (leg elevation) help to reduce postoperative pain and swelling. If the stripping is not traumatic (particularly avoiding haematomas just after stripping), most patients can walk after 4–6 hours and go home the same day, in the evening or the following day. They are advised to take regular walking exercise to activate the calf muscle pump. This procedure, performed on an out-patient basis, may save costs and bed-time in busy surgical wards. Furthermore the limited period in bed decreases the possibility of postoperative deep venous thrombosis.

Compression sclerotherapy is used to obliterate veins by injection of a sclerosing agent into the vein. The injection produces fibrotic obliteration of the collapsed veins, which is permanent. Thrombosis of the varices must be avoided as it is generally followed by recanalization and recurrence.

Method. The varicose veins to be injected are marked when the patient is standing. The patient then rests in the supine position and the sclerosing solution (0.5–1 ml of 3% sodium tetradecyl sulphate or polidocanol) is injected in the collapsed veins using a fine gauge needle. The injected venous segment is isolated by digital pressure to keep the sclerosing solution in contact with the venous walls. A local compressive bandage (i.e. an elastic adhesive bandage

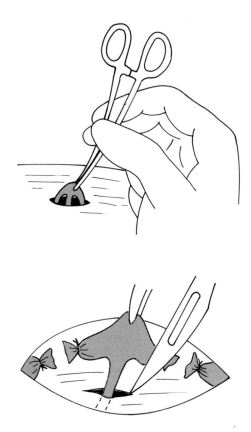

Figure 3.7. Selective ligation of an incompetent perforating vein.

such as Elastoplast or Tensoplast applied over a small cotton or paper swab) is placed on the injected area and leg compression with an elastic bandage (or graduated compression stockings in some cases) maintains the vein walls in contact until wall fibrosis has occurred. Compression prevents thrombophlebitis from developing by joining the venous walls. After a period ranging between two and four weeks the elastic bandage may be removed. During the first session it is wise to inject only a reduced quantity of the sclerosing agent to evaluate possible local and generalized reactions and the patient's compliance. Then several varices may be injected in one single session.

Sclerotherapy is a typical out-patient procedure, is less expensive than surgical treatment, and when injection is effective the cosmetic result is the best of any method. In experienced hands complications (painful injections around the vein, skin pigmentation, lesions or ulcerations) are uncommon and easy to treat. It has been observed that short term results of injection sclerotherapy are as good as surgery but long-term follow-up indicates a higher rate of recurrency with sclerotherapy in comparison with surgery.

However, the two methods are not strictly comparable, as they basically have different indications. It is very important to be able to use both methods according to the stage of venous disease and to the needs of the individual patient.

Ideally compression sclerotherapy is more effective for smaller varices and dilated superficial veins, for below-knee perforators and residual or recurrent veins after surgery. Sclerotherapy above the knee is often less satisfactory because compression tends to be less effective proximally. Surgical treatment (ligation) gives better results for venous sites with severe incompetence such as the sapheno-femoral junction, large perforators, or large varicose veins in direct connection with the main saphenous trunk.

Definition of minor and major incompetence. Severe superficial venous incompetence is demonstrated by ambulatory venous pressure (AVP) or APG. The AVP tracing indicates that the refilling time (RT) after exercise is very fast (shorter than 14 sec) in severe incompetence of the long saphenous vein. The exclusion of this vein with a cuff normalizes the RT (and AVP), indicating that ligation or stripping of the saphenous vein should be effective in normalizing the AVP and RT. Any incompetent venous site which modifies the RT and AVP can be defined as a site of *major incompetence (MI)*.

These MI sites are better treated with surgery as results are immediate and permanent. Varicose veins which do not modify the AVP–APG tracing or only moderately modify the RT without altering the AVP should be considered as a site of minor incompetence (Min) which is not associated with very important reflux. These Min sites are usually effectively treated with compression sclerotherapy, with long-lasting results. Most residual veins after surgery do not modify AVP–APG tracings and therefore are generally treated successfully with sclerotherapy. An MI venous site is therefore defined by the presence of reflux which modifies the AVP and RT (i.e. at the sapheno-femoral junction). This is generally seen by colour duplex as a huge reflux in the vein lasting more than 3 sec (at a compression-release manoeuvre) when the patient is standing.

As an alternative to sclerotherapy and standard surgery, venous incompetence can be treated with small skin incisions (1–2 mm) along the vein using small hooks to pull out and remove the veins (Muller–Georgiev method). No stitches are used, with excellent cosmetic results. The method, used on an out-patient basis, is very effective for veins associated with a low level of venous hypertension.

Sclerotherapy during surgery. Sclerotherapy can be also used during surgery to sclerose venous segment distal or proximal to ligation of major trunks (Figure 3.6), or to sclerose small, distal venous segments. This type of sclerotherapy is very effective as venous recanalization is blocked by ligation. The period of elastic compression of the sclerosed venous trunk after ligation is shorter (1–2 weeks) as there is no proximal reflux.

Treatment of small varicosities (less than 2 mm in diameter) and venous telangectasias. This cannot be considered a disease or a clinical problem as no signs or symptoms are associated with "capillary" veins. These small vein dilatations can be effectively treated with sclerotherapy using a fine gauge needle. When the most important (usually central) of the small dilated veins is injected, all the veins in the area may disappear. Low concentration (0.2–0.5%) polidocanol (or some other diluted sclerosing agent) is used and local compression is maintained for a few days. In the case of associated varicose veins it is better to treat the larger varicose veins first and the small teleangectasias after a few days. As a simple rule, for *small vein sclerotherapy* the smaller venous dilatations (veins of 1 mm diameter of less) are treated with 0.5–1% sclerosing agent and one week of compression; 1–2% solution and two weeks of compression (stockings) are used for veins between 1 and 2 mm. For veins of diameter greater than 3 mm, a 2–3% solution and 3 weeks or more of compression are used. Very small, red–pink vein dilatations are more difficult to treat than the "blue" venular teleangectasias. Short and long term results after treatment tend to be much better with the "blue" venous teleangectasias. Being a very lucrative part of venous treatment, the management of these small veins may be proposed with some "new techniques". However, no serious, reliable data is available concerning the treatment of these small vein dilatations with methods such as phothotherapy or laser.

Results and Prognosis

As varicose veins are a chronic disease, seldom treated with one single intervention, recurrence or the development of some new dilated or incompetent venous segments is common even in patients treated correctly. Even after the most appropriate treatment some varicose veins may recur in 5–15% of patients. Therefore it is a good policy to see patients regularly (i.e. every year) after the intervention (surgery and/or sclerotherapy) to identify residual or newly developing varicosities and treat them (usually with sclerotherapy) before they become enlarged and cause a new cosmetic or clinical problem. Whenever possible, *selective, limited or nondestructive surgery* should be used. New surgical techniques (i.e. perforate-invaginated stripping using a short semirigid stripper according to Goren) tend to treat more selectively only the varicose venous segment (Figure 3.8).

Noninvasive investigation is very useful for localizing venous insufficiency and the several anatomic and pathologic, possible variations observed particularly in the superficial venous system (Figure 3.9). A common cause of important recurrence is incorrect ligation of tributaries of the greater saphenous system at the sapheno-femoral junction (see Figures 3.1 and 3.9). Failure to ligate the most important incompetent perforators may also cause severe recurrence. Some important recurrences may be due to high venous pressure in the deep system trasmitted to the superficial system. In this case deep venous hypertension must be evaluated and possibly controlled or corrected. Signs and symptoms disappear or are reduced after any correct intervention and the cosmetic results are generally very good when the correct diagnosis is made and the best treatment applied. The debate between advocates of traditional surgery (such as stripping), out-patient-based, surgical techniques or sclerotherapy is more or less irrelevant, as in a good *venous clinic*, offering a complete diagnostic and treatment service, all methods of investigations and treatment should be equally and effectively made available to satisfy all clinical needs and patients' requirements. It is important to consider that one single method does not cover all the possible clinical situations and therefore

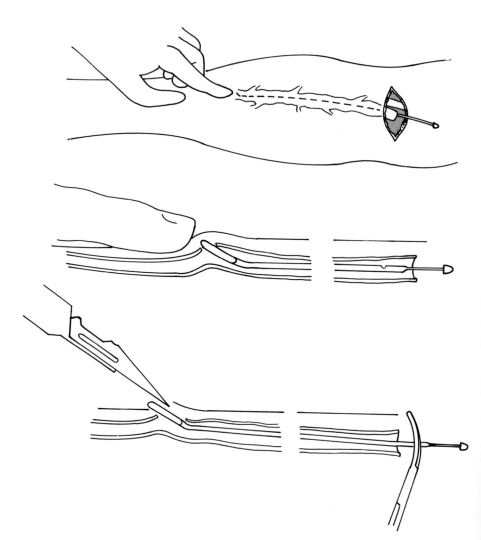

Figure 3.8. Selective stripping (perforate-invaginated stripping) using a semirigid stripper (Goren and Yellin).

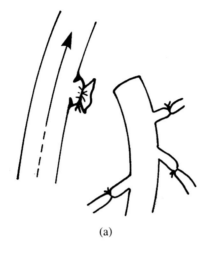

(a)

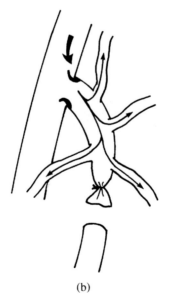

(b)

Figure 3.9. Failure in ligating the long saphenous vein close to the femoral vein (a) and all collateral veins close to the junction is an important cause of recurrence (b).

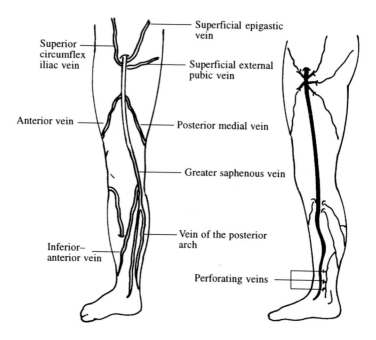

Superior circumflex iliac vein

Superficial epigastic vein

Superficial external pubic vein

Anterior vein

Posterior medial vein

Greater saphenous vein

Vein of the posterior arch

Inferior–anterior vein

Perforating veins

Figure 3.10. Stripping may still be used to remove large varicosities but after stripping many venous trunks remain.

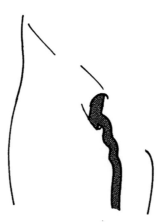

Figure 3.11. Many veins are dilated and not varicose and a simple ligation of the sapheno-femoral junction may correct the incompetence.

it is essential to be skilled and experienced in all forms of treatment. Stripping may still be used to remove large varicosities. However, it must be remembered that after stripping, many clinically significant venous trunks remain (Figure 3.10) and that some form of treatment should be provided for those veins (i.e. sclerotherapy, ligation). Finally, it is important to note that many veins are just dilated and not varicose yet. In these cases a simple ligation/section of the sapheno-femoral junction (Figure 3.10) may correct the incompetence and the vein may recover its shape and tone. Therefore in patients with dilated (more than varicose) veins a more conservative approach must always be considered.

CHAPTER 4

SUPERFICIAL THROMBOPHLEBITIS

Diagnosis

- Presence of a tender, indurated, palpable cord along a superficial vein. The long saphenous vein or one of its tributaries, most often below the knee, are generally affected.
- Redness and heat in the affected area.
- The limb is not swollen unless there is deep venous thrombosis.
- Deep venous thrombosis may develop if the tail of the thrombus extends into a deep vein.
- Systemic signs (low grade fever and, rarely, an increased white cell count).

Introduction and General Considerations

Superficial thrombophlebitis (STP) is a poorly understood and often neglected clinical condition. It is commonly seen in older patients often in association with malignancy. It usually follows minor trauma to a superficial varicose vein, resulting in localized thrombosis and in a palpable cord along the line of the affected vein. The causes of STP include:

(1) Mechanical or chemical trauma or injury (i.e. venous infusion, catheter introduction, etc);
(2) Radiation injury;
(3) Bacterial or fungal infections;
(4) Blood disorders;
(5) Immune reactions;
(6) Malignancy;
(7) Buerger's disease.

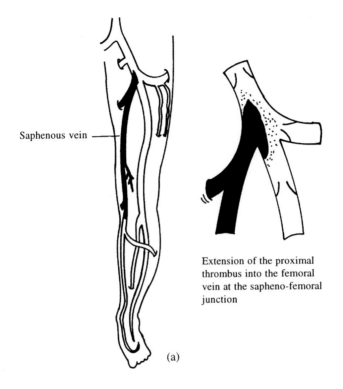

Saphenous vein

Extension of the proximal
thrombus into the femoral
vein at the sapheno-femoral
junction

(a)

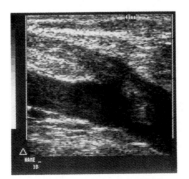

(b)

Figure 4.1. (a) Extension of the proximal thrombus into the femoral vein at the sapheno-femoral junction. After ligation and section of the long saphenous vein the thrombus is removed at the level of the sapheno-femoral junction. (b) Ultrasound image of a thrombus extending into the femoral vein.

In the upper extremities drug abuse and catheters are common causes of SVT. Although it appears to be inflammatory in nature, the background is usually noninfective. In thrombophlebitis the thrombus adheres to the vein wall and the distal venous segment tends to propagate distally. The proximal end of the thrombus may occasionally propagate into the deep venous system directly, i.e. at the sapheno-femoral junction (Figure 4.1) or through an incompetent perforating vein. The thrombus may embolize to the lungs, although this event is rare. Furthermore, the dimension of the embolus being very limited, signs and symptoms of pulmonary embolization are very rarely observed. STP is often resolved spontaneously with elevation of the affected limb and, when rarely septic, with antibiotic therapy. As noted above, progression to DVT, PE and the postphlebitic syndrome occurs only rarely. The inflammatory reaction usually takes between two and six weeks to subside (according to the extension of the process), but the thrombosed vein may be palpable and tender for months.

Attacks of STP in an incompetent superficial system with large varicose veins may be repeated (in the same or in other venous segments) unless the varicose veins are treated.

Diagnosis

STP is often seen in patients with large varicose veins and often in pregnancy. It is usually easy to diagnose, due to the superficial nature of the disease. The thrombosed veins feel like cords or a chain of nodules which are much warmer and redder than the surrounding areas.

In doubtful cases a simple test to diagnose STP consists in elevating the affected leg. If elevation does not reduce the volume of the veins as promptly seen with simple varicose veins, the veins are thrombosed.

The process most commonly used involves the long saphenous vein and its tributaries and tends to remain localized. STP is generally accompanied by local pain and induration, heat, tenderness and redness along the course of the vein. The patient may be febrile and have leukocytosis. Usually there is no oedema or swelling of the extremity, although occasionally pain and immobilization may cause differences in the size of the two limbs due to stasis and swelling.

Noninvasive investigations are generally used to rule out deep venous thrombosis. B-mode ultrasound imaging is mainly useful for excluding deep venous thrombosis. It indicates STP when the superfial veins are not compressible under the ultrasound probe. B-mode scanning is useful for showing the level and extension of the superficial thrombus and to follow up its evolution (extension or reduction).

Invasive investigations, e.g. ascending venography, are nowadays seldom performed, due to the efficacy of ultrasound studies.

Differential diagnosis. STP is generally easy to diagnose. In the obese patient STP may be confused with cellulitis. The line of redness along the affected vein makes the distinction between the two conditions easier. Other acute inflammatory conditions, e.g. panniculitis or insect bites, erythema nodosum and lymphangitis, may be confused with acute superficial thrombophlebitis. Deep venous thrombosis can occasionally be confused with superficial STP. Oedema and swelling are often associated with deep venous thrombosis while the indurated superficial venous cord is typical of STP.

In rare cases deep venous thrombosis and STP coexist when the superficial phlebitis extends into the deep system via the communicating veins or at the sapheno-femoral junction. Chills and high fever suggest infection or suppuration in the involved vein (septic thrombophlebitis).

Staphylococcus aureus is the micro-organism most frequently observed.

Treatment

Nonsurgical treatment may be used in most cases. Patients are treated with limb elevation, local heat therapy, analgesics for pain, and nonsteroidal anti-inflammatory drugs. Patients should be followed up every few days to ensure that there is no proximal extension up the thigh or into the deep venous system. Should there be any sign of extension into the deep system with thrombosis, in-patient care with intravenous heparin followed by oral anticoagulant treatment must be carried out. Subcutaneous heparin or LMWH may be used to prevent the extension of STP to the superficial or deep venous system if the definitive treatment (surgery) is delayed.

Surgical treatment may be used in patients with recent thrombosis and fresh clots in the veins. Under local anaesthesia the area is incised with a small blade and the clot removed by compressing the vein and squeezing out the thrombus. A compression bandage is used and elevation applied on an out-patient basis. The removal of the thrombus will speed up healing, reducing inflammation and pain in the area.

With more severe cases involving varicose veins these can be managed surgically, admitting patients and treating them on an elective basis. In STP extending above mid-thigh toward the sapheno-femoral junction, pulmonary embolism is rare but possible. Ligation and division of the saphenous vein at the junction and removal of the phlebitic veins and associated tributaries are indicated. Any extension of the thrombus into the common femoral vein should be removed via the opening of the long saphenous vein at the sapheno-femoral junction. STP of the short saphenous vein should likewise be managed by ligating the short saphenus vein at entry into the popliteal vein also removing the affected venous segment.

When the vein is infected (septic thrombophlebitis), the appropriate antibiotic treatment should be given, and the phlebitic segment should be removed to avoid diffusion of the bacterial infection into the bloodstream with a high risk of septic complications.

STP Without Varicose Veins

Thrombophlebitis migrans is observed when a short segment of the vein (often in the arm) becomes phlebitic. This problem is often associated with the presence of tumours (such as mucin-secreting carcinoma involving the body and tail of the pancreas, stomach, lung, breast and colon). Also, collagen disease and myelo-proliferative diseases are associated with thrombophlebitis. The definition of thrombophlebitis migrans indicates that the phlebitis resolves in one area and begins in another. These attacks of phlebitis may occur years before carcinoma is diagnosed in any of the above-mentioned organs. There is also a higher incidence of associated deep venous thrombosis.

Episodes of STP have been observed in *Bechet's syndrome*. This disorder is a multisystem disease consisting of orogenital ulcerations, vascular manifestations, superficial thrombophlebitis and recurrent iriditis. The *Budd–Chiari syndrome* may be associated.

Buerger's disease (thromboangiitis obliterans) may be defined as a segmental obliterative disease of small and medium size arteries of the extremities. It is seen in young adults and has a strong association with cigarette smoking. Up to one third of cases present with recurrent, migratory superficial thrombophlebitis. Periodic attacks of STP in young, heavy smokers suggest the possibility of Buerger's disease.

In *Mondor's disease* an STP in the upper extremities or over the chest wall is observed. It is usually seen in young adults and may have an association with smoking. A palpable cord is found in the vicinity of the inflamed vein. It may be associated with an underlying chronic pulmonary infection. The disease runs a self-limiting course and the treatment is symptomatic.

Conclusions

Most cases of STP resolve spontaneously, within a few weeks, with simple symptomatic treatment. Pulmonary embolism is uncommon, as vein wall inflammation produces adherence of the thrombus. In more severe cases noninvasive investigations are important in excluding the extension of the phlebitis into the deep venous system. Recurrent STP and/or the presence of large varices which may cause new episodes of thrombophlebitis are indications for the removal (i.e. stripping) or ligation of the varicose veins.

In the absence of varicose veins the occurrence of STP may be the first sign of a systemic disorder.

CHAPTER 5

SUBCLAVIAN AND AXILLARY VENOUS THROMBOSIS

Diagnosis

- Swelling of the entire arm.
- Collateral veins over anterior chest wall.
- Swelling and pain are worse during exercise.
- History of unusual effort or muscular activity of upper extremity.
- Colour duplex or phlebography may indicate obstruction of a proximal vein at the thoracic outlet.

Introduction and General Considerations

The anatomy of the subclavian, axillary-brachial veins and of the superficial veins of the arms are shown in Figure 5.1.

Subclavian and axillary vein thrombosis (SAVT) accounts for only 1–2% of detected cases of deep venous thrombosis. The relatively low incidence of subclavian thrombosis is thought to be due to the short length of these veins and the relative absence of venous stasis compared to the lower limbs. By aetiology subclavian and axillary venous thrombosis may be classified into three groups (Table 5.1).

SAVT associated with temporary or permanent intraluminal devices implanted for diagnostic or therapeutic purposes account for 30% of cases of subclavian and axillary venous thrombosis. Even in asymptomatic patients evidence of previous thrombosis is found in up to 40% of veins prior to a second procedure for vascular access. The incidence of thrombosis is reduced

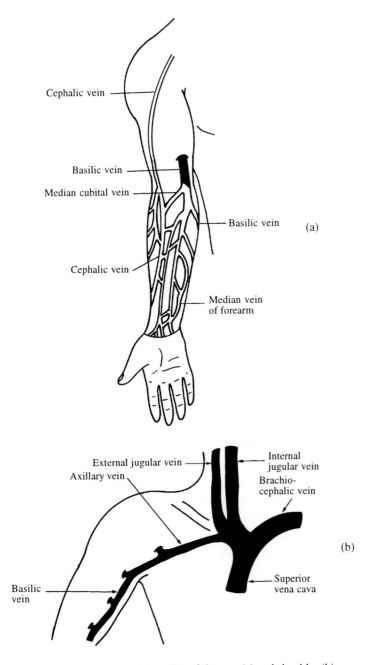

Figure 5.1. Anatomy of the veins of the arm (a) and shoulder (b).

Table 5.1. Aetiologic factors in the pathogenesis of subclavian and axillary venous thrombosis (C Fisher, DTA Hardman, 1995).

Iatrogenic: A. *In situ* device B. Previous device		
Spontaneous: Thoracic outlet syndrome		
Medical: A. Hypercoagulable state	congenital malignancy	occult overt
B. Low flow	stasis	cardiac failure
	external compression	retrosternal goitre aneurism malignancy
C. Vein injury		trauma drug injection post-radiotherapy

by low dose anticoagulation (subcutaneous low dose heparin or mini-dose warfarin).

Spontaneous or effort-related SAVT, termed the *Paget–von Schroetter syndrome*, is responsible for 30–40% of cases. This syndrome may present as a compression of a single structure or combination of the subclavian artery, the subclavian vein or the T1 root of the brachial plexus as these structures cross the first rib. The subclavian vein is affected in isolation in 10% of cases. Chronic intermittent compression produces damage to the vein wall and results in fibrosis with stenosis and/or thrombosis. A recent increase in muscle bulk may also precipitate obstruction.

The aetiological factors present in the remainder of the patients are heterogeneous but can be characterized by the presence of at least one of the main factors responsible for venous thrombosis (alteration of blood flow, or coagulation or vessel wall abnormalities). Systemic hypercoagulable states include deficiency of Protein C, Protein S, antithrombin III, lupus inhibitor, antiphospholipid syndrome or anticardiolipin antibodies. Possibly the most common of these will prove to be the recently described abnormalities in Factor V resulting in resistance to activated Protein C. Such conditions, although uncommon, should be suspected in younger patients with a history of unprecipitated thrombotic episodes. Malignancy (with or without radiation fibrosis) accounts for 20% of subclavian vein thrombosis and should always be considered in the differential diagnosis even if the initial findings are negative.

Acquired post-thrombotic states may develop with malignancy, occult or overt.

Physical examination of these patients must include specific assessment of the breast, pelvis and rectum as well as lymph nodes, specifically the supraclavicular lymp nodes. Basic investigations should include a chest X-ray. CT scanning of the thorax and abdomen may be considered. Low flow states in severe congestive cardiac failure may also cause subclavian and axillary venous thrombosis. The vessel can be injured in a variety of ways in addition to the thoracic outlet syndrome. Direct injury by adjacent structures such as fractured bones (i.e. clavicle, scapula, first rib or proximal humerus) may occur. Anterior dislocation of the humerus can also compress the axillary vein. Other rare congenital causes of axillary vein compression include abnormal insertions of biceps brachii and latissimus dorsi muscle. Damage to intima can result from hypertonic intravenous solutions, illicit drug injection and inclusion of the subclavian vein in a radiotherapy field.

Clinical Presentation

The mode of clinical presentation of SAVT depends upon the underlying aetiology. In the medical and iatrogenic groups, the patient's demographics represent the underlying disease process. The left arm is relatively more commonly involved by catheters as a consequence of the longer intravenous course of the foreign body and the angulation at the termination of the left brachiocephalic vein. SAVT may develop clinically some time after the removal of the catheter. The thoracic outlet syndrome is more common in heavily built males (male-to-female ratio = 3.5:1) and thin younger females, and the right arm is affected more frequently than the left (R:L = 2:1), reflecting the dominance of the right hand in the population. The syndrome may present acutely 24–72 hours after an initiating event such as trauma or a repetitive unusual exercise, or may appear spontaneously. The thrombosis may remain asymptomatic and only be discovered when the vessel cannot be reaccessed or when screening prior to reaccess or as an accidental finding.

The typical symptoms of SAVT include an aching pain or discomfort in the arm, with an associated heaviness made worse by activity and relieved by rest and elevation. Swelling of the whole arm and stiff fingers due to nonpitting oedema may extend to the chest wall and may be so extensive that swelling of the breast may occur. The dependent parts of the affected limb may have the mottled, cyanotic appearance of venous stasis. Veins are prominent in the hand and forearm with distended superficial veins evident over the shoulder and the anterior chest wall. A palpable, tender thrombosed cord may be present in the axillary or basilic vein. Distension of the ispilateral jugular vein suggests a more proximal thrombosis.

Rarely, *phlegmasia cerulea dolens* and *venous gangrene* may complicate the presentation in patients with severe intercurrent medical problems and are frequently an agonal event.

Pulmonary emboli occur in some 25% of cases and may occasionally be significant, with long term pulmonary damage and pulmonary hypertension. The implanted prosthetic device (usually venous access devices) may also be infected. Fungal and opportunistic infection are particularly difficult to diagnose and treat. If embolization occurs metastatic infection may follow.

Diagnosis

The diagnosis is usually apparent on clinical grounds but should be confirmed objectively. Colour duplex scanning is very effective (Figure 5.2) and has the advantage of being noninvasive although scanning around catheters is sometimes difficult. Phlebography is used only for the most complex cases or when duplex scanning is not available. Injection of contrast may often be made via existing catheters, haemodialysis access or peripheral veins. CT scanning with contrast and MRI or CT have also been used to diagnose subclavian thrombosis.

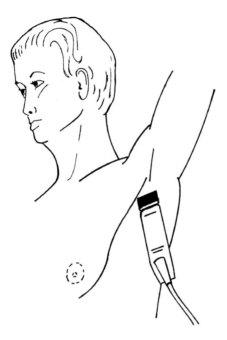

Figure 5.2. Colour duplex of the axillary vein. Position of the probe.

Treatment

Catheter-related thrombosis. Removal of the catheter and systemic anticoagulation generally relieves symptoms. The contralateral side is still usually accessible. However, when extensive or multiple episodes of thrombosis have occurred, neither the subclavian nor the jugular vein may be accessible. The loss of venous or haemodialysis access may be critical for patient care. Delay in removal with extension of the thrombosis may occur in an attempt to preserve the access. Attempted new access may entail significant additional risk for the patients, but other routes, including tranfemoral, transiliac and caval via a translumbar approach, have been described.

Subclavian vein thrombosis due to previous or current cannulation may develop proximal to a functioning arteriovenous access. The symptoms are more severe than usual, due to the high inflow pressure, and optimum treatment would involve closure or removal of the fistula. Thrombolysis or venous stenting may also be attempted and venous bypass has been performed with salvage of the access and relief of symptoms.

Thrombosis associated with medical conditions. Treatment consists generally of anticoagulation when not contraindicated. The nature of the underlying medical condition usually determines the overall outcome and treatment of the patient, and more aggressive methods of treatment are not necessarily appropriate. However, balloon dilatation and stenting of the subclavian and brachiocephalic veins have been performed for thrombosis due to malignant external compression.

Thoracic outlet syndrome. The diagnosis of the thoracic outlet syndrome may not always be clear with many patients presenting with an apparently spontaneous thrombosis. In the absence of identifiable precipitating medical conditions, patients are usually presumed to have a thoracic outlet syndrome. Although the established conservative treatment is anticoagulation with heparin, higher rates of vein patency and reduced rates of long term symptoms of venous hypertension are said to occur when more aggressive approaches are used, such as excision of the first rib through cervical or transaxillary approaches. However, no prospective randomized trials have been conducted.

Thrombolytic therapy using urokinase, streptokinase or t-PA has been demonstrated to be effective in clearing subclavian thrombosis and seems to be more effective than heparin alone. Even higher rates of patency are claimed to result when thrombolysis is combined with surgical decompression of the vein (first rib excision) and, if required, vein repair (venous patch or balloon venoplasty with or without stenting).

Venous *thrombectomy* is occasionally performed to relieve venous obstruction and to preserve valvular integrity. However, the operation is seldom successful, as rapid postoperative rethrombosis occurs in most cases if the predisposing extraluminal compression is not removed simultaneously.

Prognosis

Rapid recovery from the initial symptoms occurs in most young patients, but residual signs and symptoms may occur in some 50–80% of patients treated conservatively. Usually the acute swelling and arm pain disappear within 1–3 weeks. Some patients have persistent or recurrent symptoms such as swelling, numbness, easy tiredness, and episodes of recurrent superficial phlebitis may be observed. All symptoms are usually made worse by exercise. As a result many authors advise an aggressive approach with early thrombolysis and first rib resection.

CHAPTER 6

CHRONIC VENOUS INSUFFICIENCY AND THE POSTPHLEBITIC SYNDROME

Diagnosis

- Previous history of deep venous thrombosis may be present.
- Chronic oedema, hyperpigmentation, skin induration and lipodermato-sclerosis of skin of the distal leg and ankle.
- Ulceration, especially above the medial malleolus, is the final event.
- Secondary varicose veins.

Introduction and General Considerations

The principal late complication of deep vein thrombosis is chronic venous stasis, and most patients with serious problems have originally had iliofemoral thrombosis. Persistent obstruction from incomplete recanalization of the thrombosed veins, destruction of the valves, and reflux through incompetent perforator veins causes high pressure in the superficial venous system. Chronic venous insufficiency (CVI) is a widespread, serious and often underestimated problem. It affects some 0.5% of the UK and USA populations. Female patients appear to be affected twice as much as males. The mean age of presentation for females is 55 years and 10% of patients are hospitalized at least once for recurrent thrombosis, cellulitis, lipodermatosclerosis, venous ulceration for different forms of treatment including surgery. It has been calculated that two million workdays are lost in the USA each year for complications caused by chronic deep venous insufficiency.

The majority of cases possibly are — or are considered to be — late sequelae of DVT, hence the term *postphlebitic syndrome*, which is generally used to define (although not always correctly) CVI.

Other factors, such as congenital absence or incompetence of the valves, congenital or chronic dilatation of the deep venous system, may also be the initial cause of chronic deep venous insufficiency. A population with primary vein valvular incompetence has been identified. It is possible that some of the patients thought to have silent deep venous thrombosis suffer instead from this syndrome. This abnormal anatomical situation may be associated with venous stasis and a higher incidence of deep venous thrombosis.

The specific morphological causes of chronic deep venous insufficiency in a particular patient may not be determinant when medical or conservative management is successful. However, when direct reconstruction of the deep venous system is planned, surgery must be performed on the basis of a clear understanding of the particular disease process and its anatomy.

The acute onset of deep venous insufficiency associated with signs of obstruction in previously healthy patients, particularly the elderly, suggests the need to search for extrinsic causes of compression, such as pelvic tumours, aneurysms, etc.

Pathophysiology of CVI

Iliofemoral venous thrombosis is considered to be the most common precursor of deep venous insufficiency. A clear history of iliofemoral thrombosis is found in 20–87% of patients with deep venous insufficiency, while many patients may have had silent episodes in the past. However, a group of patients with chronic venous disease due to primary valvular incompetence, agenesis or dysfunction have been identified, although the precise percentage of such patients is unknown. It has been observed that up to 86% of patients with a previously documented deep venous thrombosis may be expected to develop a venous ulcer if followed for 10 years. The evolution of the sequelae of deep venous thrombosis is still unclear and confusing. It has been observed that about 25% of patients with thrombosis extending above the knee level may not develop symptoms for many years (5–15). In the months that follow thrombosis, recanalization of the veins restores patency but competency is often lost as thrombosis and the healing process partially or totally alter the involved valves and their function. Venous valves distal to the thrombus are thought to dilate sequentially as the proximal incompetent venous segment transmits an abnormally high hydrostatic pressure to the next distal valve. The increase in intravenous pressure is eventually transmitted to the perforating veins, which dilate with loss of competency and reversal of venous flow. This combination of progressive deep and perforating venous incompetence often leads to CVI. *Incompetent perforators* have been considered to be an important pathologic factor in some 60% of patients with CVI. Deep and perforating valve incompetence together are also considered important factors in symptomatic deep venous insufficiency. In addition, it has been observed that popliteal vein incompetence correlates best with signs and symptoms of deep venous insufficiency and ulcer recurrence after treatment. As a consequence of chronic deep venous insufficiency determining chronic venous hypertension, the increased venous pressure is transmitted to the venules and the microcirculation and the pathological process affects the skin and subcutaneous tissues. In chronic venous insufficiency the capillary network is altered, with elongation and dilatation of the capillaries, which assume a glomerulus-like appearance with thickening of the capillary wall (Figure 6.1).

In association with the morphological changes in the microcirculation, increased skin flux may be observed (by laser Doppler flowmetry) in the perimalleolar region (Figure 6.2) and this is associated with an increase in capillary filtration leading to oedema. The increased hydrostatic pressure in the microcirculation causes an increased chronic leakage of fluid and proteins into the interstitial space with resultant oedema, which is often the first clinical manifestation of CVI. Venous oedema initially appears in the evening, involving the ankle and lower leg, and recedes at night. It may progress with time so that the involved leg does not return to normal size after night rest. Massive swelling of the entire extremity or both legs may be seen with iliac or inferior vena cava obstruction. Other signs of CVI are stasis dermatitis, induration, local pain and ulceration usually localized in the perimalleolar region. Often associated with oedema are congestion and cyanosis of the skin leading to haemosiderin deposition and causing brown pigmentation. Stasis dermatitis and eczema are frequently associated. Chronic oedema and dermatitis lead to progressive fibrosis of the subcutaneous tissue and induration

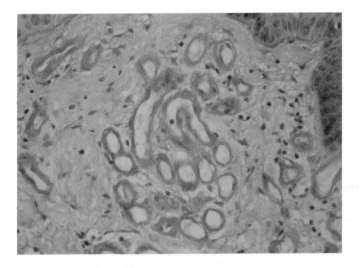

Figure 6.1. Massive dilatation of venules and capillaries in the subcutaneous tissue of a limb with venous hypertensive microangiopathy distally to a venous ulcer, in an area of venous hypertensive microangiopathy (section from the internal perimalleolar region). The dilatation and glomerulus-like aspect of the capillaries increasing the exchange surface and the thickening of the capillary wall is visible in this section.

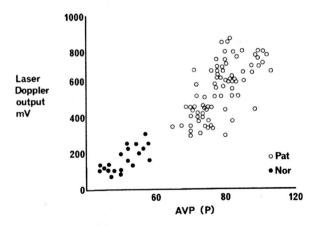

Figure 6.2. Correlation between laser Doppler flowmetry output in flux units and ambulatory venous pressure (AVP). In subjects with venous hypertension and ulcerations (circles), both venous pressure and flux are proportionally increased.

of the involved skin. These changes are usually seen in the perimalleolar area, most commonly over the medial malleolus. Perforating veins are present in this area and the incompetence of these transmits the pressure from the deep veins directly to the local microcirculation and subcutaneous tissue. An increased escape of fibrin through the microvascular network in these areas has been postulated. The excess of fibrin — and of fibrin degradation products — constitutes a dense, pericapillary "cuff" of fibrin, which an inadequate fibrinolytic system cannot clear. The fibrin wall around the more distal capillaries possibly acts as a barrier to the diffusion of gas, nutrients and metabolites, leading to cellular ischaemia and ultimately to necrosis.

However, multiple factors appear to be active in determining the microcirculatory changes observed in venous hypertensive microangiopathy. Skin oxygen tension is usually decreased in patients with CVI. The effect on the increased skin pCO_2 — in association with increased skin flux — in promoting and maintaining local vasodilatation is still unclear.

Ulceration due to chronic deep venous insufficiency is slow to heal and generally recurrent if the underlying cause of venous hypertension is not removed. In some subjects with deep venous insufficiency and severe obstruction venous claudication (a severe, bursting pain, usually of the thigh) may occur. This symptom is more common in subjects with long-standing iliofemoral obstruction, absence of collaterals and a patent distal venous system. Pain is the result of venous congestion, made worse with exercise because the increased arterial and venous flow associated with muscle activity cannot be returned to the heart at the same rate delivered. It has been observed that an increased intramuscular pressure in the anterior and deep posterior compartments and increased water content are present in the leg muscles ipsilateral to iliac vein occlusion. Therefore the pain of venous claudication appears to be mainly secondary to the acute increase in intramuscular pressure during exercise.

Diagnosis

The clinical diagnosis of CVI, with oedema, induration and ulceration, is usually made easily on history and physical examination. Differential diagnoses include congestive heart failure, chronic glomerulonephritis (these problems are associated with symmetrical swelling), chronic lymphoedema, and lipoedema. Occasionally a difficult differential diagnosis occurs between CVI and chronic lymphoedema. In chronic deep venous insufficiency oedema does not generally involve the foot and the skin and subcutaneous tissues do not show the diffuse thickening of lymphoedema with its characteristic, firm pitting oedema.

Ulceration may also result from a combination of arterial and venous disease (Table 6.1).

Table 6.1. Classification of leg ulceration (Goldstone, 1994).

(1) VASCULAR
(A) *ARTERIAL*: atherosclerosis, arteriovenous fistulas, thromboangiitis obliterans, polyarteritis nodosa, hypertension, vasospastic disease (Raynaud's).
(B) *VENOUS*: chronic venous disease, varicose veins, post-sclerotherapy, drug injection.
(C) *LYMPHATIC*: Lymphoedema.

(2) INFECTIVE
Bone (chronic osteomyelitis, fracture site), piogenic, synergistic gangrene (Meleney's ulcer), other causes (syphilis, tuberculosis, leismaniasis, leprosy, fungal disease).

(3) SYSTEMIC AND METABOLIC
Ulcerative colitis, diabetes, sickle cell anaemia, avitaminosis.

(4) NEOPLASTIC
Primary skin tumours (Kaposi's sarcoma, melanoma, squamous cell carcinoma), leukaemia, metastatic tumours.

(5) TRAUMATIC
Radiation, thermal burns, decubitus, insect bites.

(6) NEUROTROPHIC
Cord lesions; peripheral neuropathies (trauma, diabetes, tabes dorsalis, alcoholism).

Distal localization of the lesion at the toes and feet, their pale appearance, and the pain associated with them, as well as the other signs of arterial insufficiency, are useful in distinguishing between the two entities. Examination with the hand-held Doppler and measurement of ankle-brachial index will usually reveal the presence of an arterial problem. Oedema and chronic skin changes and thickening may be obstacles to accurate pulse examination, as may be the presence of calcified arteries in diabetics leading to spuriously high ankle pressures. Therefore vascular laboratory studies, both arterial and venous, are important in such situations. Whereas physical examination may reveal the presence of CVI, it is not sufficient to localize and quantify the underlying anatomic and functional defects.

In some limbs valvular incompetence may be a localized disease. Femoral veins may reflux separately, as may popliteal veins, while in some limbs incompetence may be generalized. Popliteal vein incompetence is believed to correlate most directly with the classical signs of chronic deep venous insufficiency, although femoral incompetence is the most important causal factor and some patients had proximal incompetence either localized or in conjunction with distal incompetence. If there is no apparent cause for venous thrombosis or CVI, other possibilities may be evaluated. Pelvic tumours, haemangiomas and arteriovenous fistulas may give rise to chronic, rapidly progressive venous insufficiency, as may primary valvular agenesis or post-thrombotic incompetence.

Ascending phlebography has for many years been the standard against which new diagnostic tests have been compared. Deep venous and perforator patency and/or competence can be easily demonstrated, as are postphlebitic changes and chronic obstructions. Ascending phlebography can also be performed in such a way as to define valve incompetence. If deep venous reconstructive surgery is considered, a clear definition of the state of the venous valves usually requires *descending phlebography*. Kirstner (1986) has developed a grading system for evaluating descending phlebography (Table 6.2). Decisions concerning deep venous valvular replacement or reconstruction are usually dependent on the results of such anatomic and functional assessment. Descending phlebography is a fluoroscopic, dynamic study and as such provides functional as well as anatomic data. The role of ambulatory venous pressure (AVP) and APG has been described in Chapter 2. These tests allow precise, quantitative definition of the degree of venous hypertension and are useful for following the evolution of the disease and the effect of interventions.

Table 6.2. Interpretation of descending phlebography.

Complete competence:	Does not leak during full Valsalva manoeuvre.
Satisfactory competence:	Mild leakage limited to thigh during Valsalva manoeuvre.
Moderate incompetence:	Prominent leakage into calf during Valsalva manoeuvre; retains prograde flow in iliac vein.
Severe incompetence:	Cascading retrograde flow during Valsalva manoeuvre; reflux into calf perforators.

Nonoperative Treatment of CVI

Medical management is the most common form of treatment for the majority of patients with chronic deep venous insufficiency. Education of patients is also essential. Venous disease is chronic and insidious, causing permanent damage and invalidity over years. Many physicians fail to understand the slow, progressive evolution of deep venous insufficiency and often patients do not appreciate the necessity of protracted care. The most important aim of therapy is to control venous hypertension and to avoid oedema. This may be accomplished in most patients with elastic stockings. However, in subjects with bone or joint problems, low muscular activity or any cause of low mobility of the limb, even elastic compression, may be disappointing, and active or passive motion may be crucial to ensuring improvement. Intermittent periods of leg elevation and avoidance of prolonged sitting and standing should be advised. In patients with arterial disease elastic compression is contraindicated. There is little need for elastic support above the knee, because the complications of venous insufficiency practically never extend this high. Unless the venous problem is corrected surgically, elastic compression must be used indefinitely.

Graduated elastic support is a lifelong necessity for most patients. At the moment graduated compression elastic stockings appear to provide the best support and are easier for the patient to apply than bandages. Strict adherence to the use of these stockings often prevents the consequences of chronic venous hypertension and may alleviate signs and symptoms. Knee-length stockings are usually sufficient as most of the muscular action causing venous return is in the calf and the highest venous pressure is below-knee. Stockings producing 30–40 mmHg compression at the ankle level are usually effective in controlling oedema and other signs of venous insufficiency. Ulceration is initially treated conservatively with elevation, local medication and compressive therapy, usually on an outpatient basis.

Unna's boots (semirigid zinc oxide bandages) are still used extensively but they may lead to immobilization of the ankle joint.

Selective antibiotics or antibacterial solutions are indicated only in patients with cellulitis.

Patients' allergies to local treatment and bandages must be recognised because local allergic reactions can turn small ulcerations into larger skin defects that are very difficult to heal. Eczema and dermatitis are treated keeping the skin well hydrated. Extensive ulceration with associated cellulitis may rarely require hospitalization with elevation of the leg. Skin grafting may be a necessity for some patients. Large, recurrent ulcers indicate the need for more aggressive management. The application of microcirculation techniques to evaluate venous hypertensive microangiopathy has made it possible to understand and evaluate the qualitative and quantitative changes in the microcirculation produced by elastic compression, intermittent sequential compression and drug treatment.

Surgical Management of CVI

The correction of superficial incompetence (surgery and/or sclerotherapy) aims to produce a progressive decrease in venous incompetence and venous hypertension by the interruption or obliteration of all incompetent superficial segments. This may be achieved by selective surgery after identification (by colour duplex or phlebography) of all incompetent venous sites, such as an incompetent sapheno-femoral junction or incompetent perforating veins. Often this type of surgery may be performed on an out-patient basis in repeated short sessions. Ligation of the incompetent venous sites followed by sclerotherapy of the smaller (and more distal) veins seems to be very effective. Sclerotherapy of the proximal incompetent veins appears to be less effective than sclerotherapy applied to the veins below the knee. Often one or two perforators may be identified close to the ulcer. Transcutaneous or endoscopic ligation and sclerotherapy of these perforators are useful in decreasing local venous hypertension to a level associated with faster healing. Classic operations such as the extrafascial or subfascial procedures which interrupt incompetent perforators (Figure 6.3) are now rarely used as they lead to an unacceptably high incidence of wound complications and require protracted in-patient stay. Extensive dissection can be avoided as it is possible to localize with precision incompetent perforators with colour duplex or using endoscopic methods. The new technique of subfascial endoscopic perforator surgery (SEPS) involves inserting an endoscope under the fascia through an incision in the healthy skin of the upper calf. The endoscope is then passed distally in the subfascial plane and incompetent calf perforators can be seen and interrupted. This

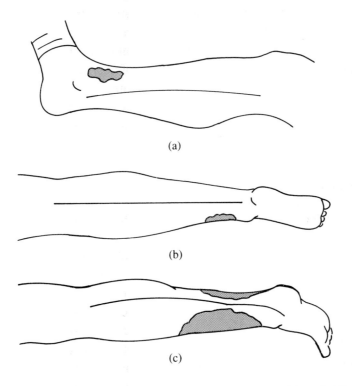

(a)

(b)

(c)

Figure 6.3. Incisions used for the Linton (a) and Felder (b) operations for ligations of perforating veins (the incision line may be modified in the case of large ulcerations). These procedures have now been replaced by direct surgery after localization of the incompetent veins by colour duplex or by endoscopic ligation of the incompetent perforating veins.

technique has been shown to produce many fewer complications than the traditional open ligation of calf perforating veins, but as yet there is no long term data relating to ulcer recurrence or guidance as to which patients should have their calf perforators ligated. In the case of associated deep and superficial venous incompetence the correction of the superficial incompetence may often be followed by a decrease in the levels of venous hypertension and by a very relevant clinical improvement (i.e. healing of ulceration). If the ulcers cannot be controlled by conservative management or if they are very large, direct surgery may be indicated. Skin grafts may be applied directly to a clean granulating ulcer. The ulcer may be also excised and a skin graft applied primarily (Figure 6.4). Recurrences are common if nothing is done to remove the diseased veins and the undelying venous hypertension. The initial operation should include ligation and/or stripping of the greater saphenous vein and ligation of incompetent perforators in the region of the ulcer. If the lesser saphenous system is involved, it should be removed as well.

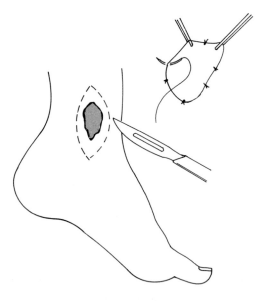

Figure 6.4. Direct surgery. Excision of the ulcerated area and skin transplant. The best results are obtained only after correction of venous incompetence and hypertension and when the ulcer is clean.

The removal of secondary varicosities of the saphenous system, except in rare instances, does not impair venous return from the extremity, unless there is deep venous obstruction.

Deep Incompetence

Direct surgical correction of chronic venous insufficiency must be reserved for well-defined patients. The important role of incompetent perforators in aggravating deep venous insufficiency when performing direct deep venous reconstruction may be overlooked. Incompetent perforators should be treated at the same time as deep venous reconstruction.

Newer procedures have been and are still being developed on the basis of a better understanding of venous pathophysiology. There remains controversy about the role of a single, competent valve at the superficial femoral vein level and about the importance of femoral incompetence versus popliteal incompetence.

Furthermore the cost of medical treatment must be balanced versus the cost and benefits of surgical procedures.

Surgery for CVI may be divided into two main categories of operative procedures:

(1) Operations to restore patency;
(2) Operations to restore venous competency.

Patency

At present there are three types of operations performed to restore patency:

(1) The Husni operation;
(2) The Palma–Dale operation and its variants;
(3) Direct reconstructions of the iliac vein and the inferior vena cava.

The *Husni operation*, or *in situ* sapheno-popliteal veno-venous bypass, is aimed at relieving obstruction of the femoral and popliteal veins using the ipsilateral saphenous vein anastomosed end-to-side to the most proximal patent deep vein, usually the popliteal. Free vein grafts can be used if the ipsilateral saphenous vein is not suitable and if the other extremity is not involved (Figure 6.5).

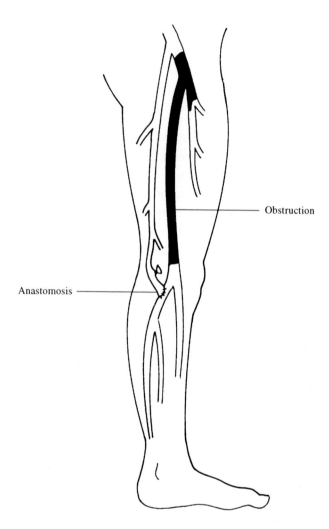

Figure 6.5. Diagram of the Husni operation (*in situ* sapheno-popliteal venous bypass). This procedure is indicated in patients with severe venous obstruction (i.e. venous claudication).

In the *Palma–Dale operation* (Figure 6.6), iliac obstruction is bypassed by the use of the contralateral saphenous vein. Patients treated with a Palma operation may have malignancies obstructing the iliac vein (43%). Of the patients over 50 years of age, many (65%) have obstruction due to pelvic cancer. The best results occur when the procedure is used to relieve extrinsic compression in which the veins themselves are structurally intact.

Unless there is an acute obstruction, before-surgery dynamic tests should clearly indicate an outflow obstruction. If patency of collaterals is of such a degree that distal venous pressures, even after exercise, are only mildly elevated, bypass grafting cannot be expected to be either necessary or successful. Externally reinforced PTFE may also be used as a crossover graft. Arteriovenous fistulas are often created at the time of operation to increase flow rates through the graft in the first postoperative days. They are usually temporary and ligated or occluded after 6–12 weeks.

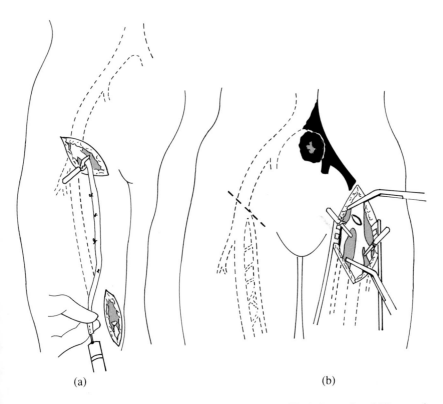

(a)   (b)

Figure 6.6. The Palma–Dale operation to bypass deep venous (iliac) obstruction. (a) Preparation of the contralateral saphenous vein; (b) preparation of the femoral vein and of the sapheno-femoral junction of the obstructed side; (c) final appearance of the bypass (an arterio-venous temporary fistula may be associated).

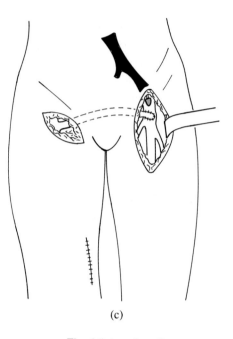

(c)

Fig. 6.6 (*continued*)

Distinct from extra-anatomic, or crosspubic, grafting are direct reconstructions of the iliac veins and the superior and inferior vena cavae, which have been performed with spiral vein grafts and with externally supported (ringed) PTFE grafts. Results are promising and it may be that direct reconstructions will prove superior to extra-anatomic grafts. Temporary arteriovenous fistulas and anticoagulation as adjuvant therapy are recommended with these procedures. Operations to restore patency are applicable to only a small minority of patients with CVI; only some 5–10% of cases of CVI are based on pure obstruction.

Competency

There are different operations aimed at restoring venous competency. They include internal and external vein valvuloplasty, transplants of valve-containing segments of the brachial vein to the femoral or popliteal levels, and vein-segment transpositions.

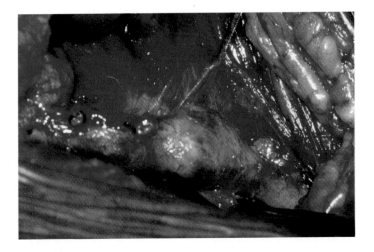

Figure 6.7. Superficial femoral vein dissected before valvuloplasty. The valve commissures are visible.

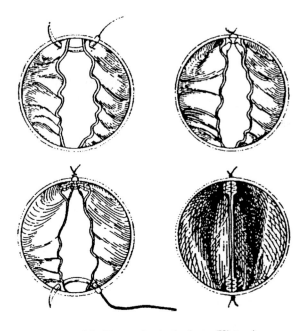

Figure 6.8. External valvuloplasty (Kistner).

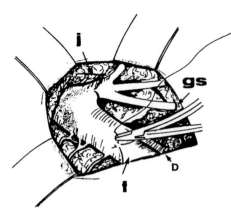

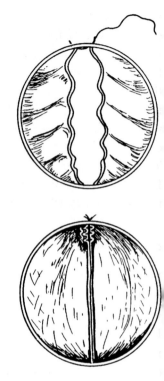

LAP is performed only on the anterior side of the superficial femoral vein after limited dissection of the anterior circumference of the vein distally to the sapheno-femoral junction (j). The limited dissection has the aim of preserving vascularization and innervation. f, superficial femoral vein; gs, greater saphenous vein; D, deep femoral vein.

The effect of LAP on approaching the vein valve cusps anteriorly is shown. The reduction in lumen of the enlarged femoral vein with anterior plication makes the femoral valve competent.

Figure 6.9.   Anterior plication of the femoral vein.

External valvuloplasty can be performed after demonstrating the presence of mobile valvular cusps in the vein by high resolution duplex scanning or phlebography (i.e. in the femoral vein). After careful no-touch dissection of the vein the valvular structure is isolated (Figure 6.7) and the valvular ring is made smaller by two opposite, continuous sutures (1–2 cm) along the cusps commissures (Figure 6.8). Valvuloplasty gives good results when the incompetence is mainly due to dilatation of the vein and the cusps are functionally intact. Some dilatation of the venous segment is often observed months after valvuloplasty and some forms of reinforcements of the venous walls around the corrected valvular ring (nets, venous cuffs). Recently a different type of *limited anterior valvuloplasty* including only the anterior surface of the valvular ring has been developed (Figure 6.9). This anterior, limited valvuloplasty is effective in making the femoral vein competent, and the limited dissection, preserving the vasa vasorum and the innervation, is not followed by dilatation of the vein. *Valvuloplasty* has also been performed recently under angioscopic vision to control the approximation of the vein cusps. Results of valvuloplasty at highly specialized centres are satisfactory. The majority of patients probably can still be treated by elastic compression. Long term results are encouraging. Venous reconstructions may therefore be performed on selected subjects when medical management is unsatisfactory.

Complications and Prognosis

Rarely, after many years, a chronic ulcer may undergo malignant transformation — a change that is not always easy to recognize. Therefore, intractable ulcers should be biopsied to evaluate the presence of a tumour. Recurrent DVT and phlebitis is more frequent than previously considered and may produce a progressive deterioration of the venous system. To avoid this complication prophylactic measures such as elastic support, periodic elevation of the legs, and avoidance of trauma and stasis-producing situations should be used.

CHAPTER 7

CHRONIC LIMB SWELLING

Swelling and oedema may be due to systemic causes or are a consequence of an increased local production and decreased removal of interstitial fluid. An imbalance develops between the filtration pressure in the proximal capillary bed and the absorptive osmotic pressure at the venous end of the capillary bed. The glomerulus-like appearance of capillaries in chronic venous insufficiency and the associated increase in the exchange surface contribute to this imbalance with accumulation of water and proteins in the interstitial fluid. The most common causes of limb oedema are indicated in Table 7.1.

Table 7.1. Clinical problems causing chronic limb swelling.

Systemic causes
Congestive heart failure, hormone/drug treatment (i.e. some calcium antagonists), nephrosis, cirrhosis, myxoedema, hypoproteinaemia

Venous
Chronic venous insufficiency
Extrinsic compression (tumours, retroperitoneal fibrosis, compression by the iliac artery on the left iliac vein)
Arteriovenous communications (AV fistulas)
Trauma (surgery, ligation of veins, caval plication, clipping)

Lymphatic
Primary limphoedema: congenital lymphoedema, early lymphoedema, late lymphoedema
Secondary lymphoedema: filariasis, infections, neoplastic disease, radiation injury, insect bites, surgical excision of lymph nodes (i.e. mastectomy), reduced limb activity (i.e. paralysis)

Primary venous or lymphatic problems, and systemic or external causes (i.e. compression by tumours), are associated with acute or chronic oedema of the limbs. In the lower limbs the problem is aggravated by gravity (standing) and partially or completely relieved by elevation.

Large protein molecules which have escaped from the capillary bed are returned to the systemic circulation via the distal lymphatic system, which is the most important draining route from the interstitial space. The decrease in the rate of removal of interstitial proteins is the most important abnormality in lymphoedema. Also, in chronic venous insufficiency the compression of the distal lymphatic branches due to oedema reduces the draining capacity of the lymphatic system. The presence of proteins in the interstitial space produces an osmotic force increasing chronic water retention, clinically evident as oedema.

In *acute venous obstruction*, oedema is due to the acutely decreased venous outflow with increased pressure and fluid filtration at venular level. The interstitial pressure increase due to oedema also excludes some of the terminal lymphatics by compression, further impairing local drainage.

In *chronic venous insufficiency (CVI)*, oedema is mainly a consequence of the chronically increased fluid and protein filtration due to the elevated venular pressure. In CVI most lymphatics still remove extracellular protein, and therefore chronic venous oedema is low in protein.

The clinical presence of oedema always indicates that interstitial fluid and lymph formation exceeds the possibile lymph resorption. Whatever the cause, chronic oedema produces comparable patterns of secondary inflammation and fibrosis due to the presence of proteins in the interstitial space. If the swelling is unilateral, the disease is generally local (i.e. post-mastectomy oedema) and the most frequent diagnostic problem is to decide whether the origin is venous or lymphatic. The presence of external compression due to tumours (usually unilateral), history of previous surgery involving lymph nodes and systemic causes of swelling (usually bilateral) must be excluded.

Occasionally, unilateral *atrophy* of one-leg (calf) muscles may confuse the clinical picture, suggesting swelling of one limb, while on the contrary the other lymb is hypotrophic. Also, *stasis due to low mobility* (i.e. following paralysis) of one limb is often associated with oedema without a real venous or lymphatic problem.

The clinical definition of swelling may be based on clinical findings in most cases. However, investigations of the venous and lymphatic systems (duplex and colour duplex, venography or lymphangiography) are very useful. In the case of sudden unexplained swelling of the lower limb, particularly in elderly patients, abdominal ultrasound, a chest radiograph and an abdominal CT scan may indicate the presence of extrinsic compression of the abdominal veins.

The treatment of swelling depends on the nature of its cause.

Unilateral oedema due to venous or lymphatic problems may generally be controlled with elastic compression and leg elevation. When physical measures are not effective, other possibilities (i.e. surgery aimed at eliminating compression or restoring patency of the deep venous system) should be considered.

Compression of the proximal segment of the left iliac vein. A special problem is unilateral swelling (usually the left distal leg and foot) in the presence of an apparently normal venous system and without any other apparent specific cause. The venous system, by ultrasound examination, appears patent, with flow phasic upon respiration and augmentation with distal manual compression of the leg. When thrombosis and any other most common causes of obstruction and incompetence have been ruled out, it is possible that a compression of the left iliac vein by the right iliac artery may be the cause of swelling.

The compression of the left iliac vein at its proximal end is usually partial and due to its anatomy. The left common iliac vein is forced forwards by the convexity of the lower lumbar vertebrae, particularly in young women, and at the same time it is crossed arteriorly by the right common iliac artery. This anatomic situation results in some degree of compression over the termination of the left common iliac vein. A filling defect on venography may be observed in some 50% of subjects with an otherwise normal iliac venogram (Figure 7.1). The compression is usually compensated for by an increase in the lateral section of the vein so that the cross-sectional area and the flow are preserved. By colour duplex the compression picture is very often less evident than with venography and it is very seldom associated with an increased venous flow velocity (indicating stenosis). It is therefore possible that venography overestimates the problems.

Noninvasive investigations (ultrasound, particularly colour duplex, are useful) and CT or MR scans may reveal and correctly localize the level of

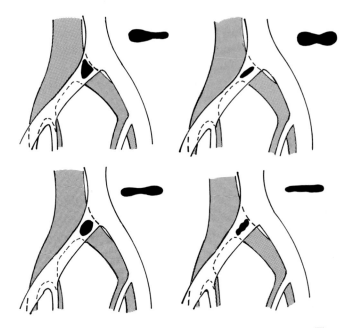

Figure 7.1. Types of iliac vein compression by the proximal right iliac artery. The compression (with the section of the vein indicated) may range from a partial compression not affecting venous flow (A) to almost complete obstruction (D).

obstruction. Venography is useful but it tends to overestimate compression as a flattened vein is not necessarily associated with flow alterations.

In some subjects the compression is more marked and sometimes associated with a band or adhesion at the proximal end of the left common iliac vein. The compression at this level has also been considered to be a possible cause of venous thrombosis which is considered to be more frequent in the left leg.

The presence of recurrent distal leg–foot oedema may require in some subjects surgical treatment or stenting of the affected segment. In some cases with severe obstruction the vein may be dissected to eliminate constricting bands or adhesions or cut and re-anastomosed end-to-end over the artery or reimplanted on the the inferior vena cava, although the results are variable. If acute thrombosis has occurred thrombolysis may be employed before surgical correction or venous stenting.

CHAPTER 8

LYMPHATICS AND LYMPHOEDEMA

Lymphatic capillaries are endothelial tubes differing from the capillaries for their high permeability to macromolecules. The lymphatic system of the lower limbs is closely associated with the venous system (Figure 8.1). The most important function of lymphatics is the removal of macromolecules from the interstitial space. Large lymphatics have some muscular wall components with

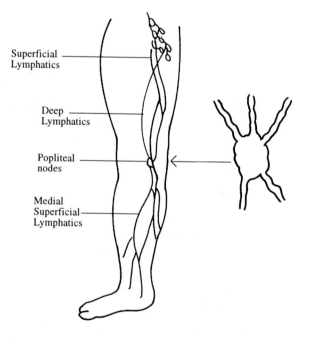

Figure 8.1. The lymphatic system of the lower limbs is closely associated with the venous system.

contracting power while endothelial valves direct lymphatic flow in a central direction. Muscular contraction during exercise and normal activity increases lymphatic flow velocity while valves prevent reflux. Lymph node stations are regularly localized along the larger lymphatics channels. Their function is filtrative and phagocytic and they also have an important immunologic function. Two to four litres of lymph (containing between 70 and 200 g of protein) enter the subclavian veins daily. The rate of lymph flow is increased in the case of muscular exercise in the early stages of venous obstruction, in inflammation and infection, and in all situations associated with vasodilatation and increased capillary permeability. The lymphatic capillaries form a superficial plexus in the superficial dermis (Figure 8.2). A deep plexus is present in the deeper dermis in the extremities and a subfascial plexus is present within the muscular compartments. Tissue fluid filtered from the capillary system is collected in dermal lymphatics and drained into subcutaneous

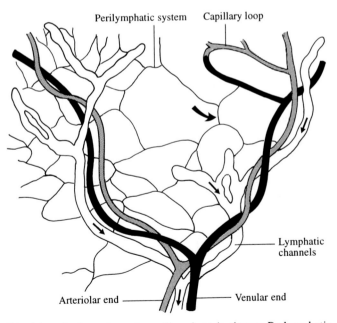

Figure 8.2. Distal lymphatic system. A capillary loop is shown. Prelymphatic spaces are indicated by arrows. They drain in the lymphatic channels which follow the course of the artery and vein.

lymphatics which follow the course of many superficial veins. Lymphatic flow drains into major regional lymphatic channels and lymph nodes. Large lymphatic vessels are usually parallel to major blood vessels.

Investigation of the Lymphatic System

Lymphangiography. Tests of pulmonary function before lymphangiography are advisable, because the contrast medium used for lymphangiography may produce a temporary diffusion barrier when it reaches the lungs, causing problems to patients with impaired lung function. An organic dye injected into the skin is drained by the the subdermal or superficial dermal lymphatic system. Local lymphatics are visualized by the presence of dye. This allows cannulation and direct injection of contrast media. The lymphangiogram usually shows lymphatics of uniform diameter branching as they approach the proximal limb. The technique is very helpful in detecting the cause of chronic swelling of the limbs and in diferentiating primary from secondary lymphoedema. Lymphangiography is also used to study lymph nodes in the retroperitoneum or mediastinum in the evaluation of some patients with lymphomas.

Lymphoscintigraphy is relatively simple, with no important side effects. After injection of a small amount of technetium 99m-labelled antimony trisulfide colloid in an interdigital space, the extremity is imaged with a gamma camera. The transport of lymph can be determined by interpretation of the imaged pattern of the lymphatic anatomy. The estimation of the appearance time of the colloid in the regional lymph nodes indicates whether lymphatic flow and channels are normal or abnormal. In lymphoedema there are abnormal patterns with delayed appearance of colloid in the proximal lymphatic stations. In patients with early chronic venous insufficiency causing oedema, a normal or moderately increased lymph transport may be seen, while in late stages of venous insufficiency an impairment in lymphatic drainage may be important in aggravating the clinical picture.

Other tests of lymphatic function. High resolution B-mode imaging of dilated (ecolucent) spaces in the subcutaneous tissue is very often associated with lymphoedema (demonstrated by lymphangiography and lymphoscintigraphy). This simple test (Figure 8.3) (Cesarone) which reveals the presence of dilated lymphatic spaces is easy and repeatable and may be

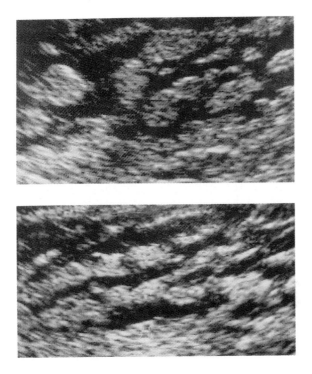

Figure 8.3. High resolution ultrasound in a case of lymphoedema. Dilated, low density (echolucent), interstitial spaces.

used to evaluate the progression of the disease or the effects of treatments (i.e. pneumatic sequential compression). In the natural history of primary lymphoedema these spaces are almost always present initially only at the dorsum of the foot and progressively extend proximally. However, these spaces are also seen (less often and less diffusely) in other clinical situations associated with oedema.

Magnetic resonance scans also demonstrate the presence of these spaces in lymphoedema.

The *spontaneous clearance of a haematoma* is assessed injecting a small amount of blood (0.4 ml in the subcutaneous tissue of the dorsum or lateral side of the foot). Repeated photos indicate the time of disappearance of the haematoma, and indirectly the lymphatic system activity. In the case of primary lymphoedema the disappearance time is prolonged.

The *ratio between the concentration of interstitial (lymphatic) fluid and the concentration of plasmatic proteins (Pflug)* can be assessed with a fine gauge needle inserted in the subcutaneous tissue of the dorsum of the foot. An increased concentration of macromolecules (proteins) in patients with lymphatic problems is usually observed due to the decreased lymphatic drainage. Also, in late chronic venous insufficiency the drainage of proteins from the interstitial space is usually impaired (Figure 8.4).

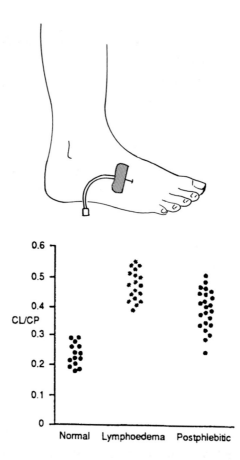

Figure 8.4. The ratio between the concentration of interstitial (lymphatic) fluid proteins and plasmatic proteins increases in patients with lymphatic problems and in severe chronic venous insufficiency.

Direct measurement of lymphatic pressure (Bollinger) indicates an increased pressure in patients with lymphoedema.

The above investigation methods are mainly used for research and are not easily available in most hospitals. Lymphangiography and lymphangioscintigraphy are the mainstays of clinical diagnosis.

LYMPHOEDEMA

Diagnosis

- Progressive swelling of one or both lower extremities. Nonpitting oedema does not respond to leg elevation.
- Recurrent episodes of lymphangitis and cellulitis are possible.
- Previous episodes of local infections are usually reported.

Introduction

Lymphoedema is caused by abnormal pooling and stagnation of interstitial lymph fluid due to either a congenital developmental abnormality of lymphatics or secondary lymphatic obstruction. Lymphoedema may be caused by several problems; however, the pathophysiologic mechanism involving obstruction of lymphatics is very similar in all.

Primary lymphoedema appears as congenital lymphoedema (early lymphoedema or late lymphoedema).

Secondary lymphoedema may be caused by filariasis, infections, neoplastic disease, radiation injury, insect bites, surgical excision of lymph nodes (i.e. mastectomy), or simply by prolonged limb inactivity (i.e. following paralysis).

Diagnosis

Primary lymphoedema may be present at birth (congenital lymphoedema) but more often becomes manifest in the teens or twenties (lymphoedema praecox or early lymphoedema). *Milroy's disease* is a form of chronic hereditary lymphoedema with very early onset (at or near birth). In a small percentage of cases, it develops after the age of 30–35 (lymphoedema tarda). It is caused by developmental lymphatic abnormalities. Lymphatic hypoplasia is present in some 50% of patients, varicose dilatation of the lymphatics in 20–30% and aplasia in less than 15% of subjects.

Regardless of the precise nature of the anatomic problem at the basis of lymphoedema the functional result is lymphatic obstruction pooling and increased interstitial pressure. The lymphatics dilate, making the valves incompetent. Since lymphatic valves are essential for stopping reflux and maintaining centripetal flow, lymphatic venous reflux aggravates stasis. The chronic presence of unremoved interstitial proteins causes fibrosis, interstitial compression and further obstruction. High levels of interstitial proteins facilitate bacterial infection. In primary lymphoedema, oedema is usually initially limited to the tissues superficial to the deep muscle fascia.

Early (lymphoedema praecox) predominantly affects young women, beginning at puberty or during adolescence. The first sign is swelling which starts as a puffiness or swelling of the dorsum of the foot or at the ankle, made worse by long periods of standing or sitting. The swelling is often unilateral at the beginning but in some subjects it may be bilateral. Some 50% of patients with primary lymphoedema eventually develop bilateral disease. The persisting oedema progresses proximally slowly. After some time (1–2 years) the entire limb may be involved. Progressively the swelling becomes marked and nonpitting. Leg elevation and bed rest become ineffective for its control. Furthermore oedema, originally soft and pitting, gradually becomes resistant to external pressure. The subcutaneous tissue becomes hypertrophic and the limb permanently enlarged. Patients often complain of the serious disfiguration and because the limb feels heavy and uncomfortable. Most patients also complain of a loss of sensation, without actual pain unless lymphangitis occurs.

Secondary lymphoedema is due to defined problems affecting the lymphatic system. Neoplastic obstruction of lymphatics is the most frequent problem. Surgical removal of lymphatics, for example during radical mastectomy or inguinal dissection, and radiotherapy are common causes. Repeated occurrence of cellulitis causes progressive closure of the lymphatics and the oedema becomes progressively more evident. In some countries filariasis is a common cause of lymphoedema. Lymphangiography and lymphoscintigraphy usually demonstrate the level and the extent of lymphatic obstruction.

Complications

As lymphoedema progresses without control or treatment, the skin and subcutaneous tissue thicken and become hyperkeratotic. Cellulitis and lymphangitis may occur, even aften minor trauma, and are the most frequent complications. Swelling, erythema, pain and occasionally systemic signs of infection may be present. With an impaired lymphatic system the infection tends to diffuse more rapidly along the lymphatic channels. This is indicated by red streaks in the skin. Streptococcus is frequently present in these types of infection.

Lymphangiosarcoma, an uncommon neoplasm originating from the lymphatic endothelium, may occur as a late complication of chronic lymphoedema (most commonly with postmastectomy lymphoedema of the arm). It tends to spread rapidly and has a very poor prognosis. This tumour appears as multiple macular or papular lesions in the skin or subcutaneous tissue. The lesion may form a large ulcerating mass.

Differential Diagnosis

Lymphoedema is easily differentiated from systemic diseases as oedema is bilateral, soft and pitting (i.e. congestive heart failure, cirrhosis or nephrosis). Lymphoedema is also easily differentiated from chronic deep venous insufficiency with noninasive investigations (showing a normal venous system) and because very often venous dilatations and varicosities are present in venous disease. Furthermore, the swelling of lymphoedema is generally painless, rubbery and nonpitting and decreases little if at all with leg elevation or night rest. In chronic venous insufficiency the oedema is soft and pitting initially, but in late stages is more firm, associated with skin pigmentation, stasis dermatitis and evenually ulceration. Recurrent lymphangitis and cellulitis are more frequent in lymphoedema. Some degree of lymphatic impairment or real lymphoedema may exist in patients with a postphlebitic limb. The differentiation is based on noninvasive investigation and occasionally on lymhoscintigraphy (rarely on lymphangiography).

Obesity Lymphoedema

Some degree of lymphatic impairment and oedema is also often observed in very obese subjects and readily diagnosed as lymphoedema. However, these conditions are partially or totally reversible with a significant loss of weight and exercise. On the contrary, most patients with true lymphoedema are very rarely obese.

Control and Treatment of Lymphoedema

Chronic and careful control of the oedema is the key to limiting the number of complications and the progression of lymphoedema. The prevention of recurrent infection is also very important. When oedema control and treatment are planned and used in the very early stages, before fibrosis occurs, the results are satisfactory.

(1) *Physical treatment and nonoperative management.* Oedema in most patients with early lymphoedema is effectively controlled with physical measures. The objective of any treatment is to control the development of oedema and lymph formation with elevation, periodically during the day, and at night (20–30 cm elevation of the distal leg). Elastic compression stockings are used as much as possible during the day. The stocking should include the entire leg. Pneumatic, sequential compression is very useful. It is used for 2–3 hours daily or at night. Lymphatic sequential compression devices are effective (but expensive). Simple one-chamber devices are also effective. The best results are obtained with sequential compression applied in the evening before or during sleep. The restriction of dietary sodium may be considered in some patients, but the use of diuretics in true lymphoedema is very questionable. Skin and foot care is very important for preventing infections, cellulitis and lymphangitis. If infections recur often, patients must be treated with specific antibiotics bearing in mind that the prevalent organism causing infection is usually a streptococcus.

Strenuous, continuous physical exercise in young subjects is very beneficial when possible. Devices (*ovens*) increasing local temperature promote interstitial protein degradation and, in association with manual lymph drainage, may be effective. The degraded proteins are removed faster from the interstitial tissue, the rate of progression of the oedema decreases and the skin becomes softer. However, this type of treatment has not been proven widely and there is no safety data indicating whether it may further damage the lymphatic system. *Repeated manual lymphatic drainage* when performed by expert and specialized staff may be very effective in the early phases.

(2) *Surgical treatment* is indicated only in a very limited number (10–15%) of patients. Indications for surgery are:

- Very impaired limb function due to deformity (mainly excess in size and weight);
- Severe pain;
- Repeated episodes of infections;
- Neoplastic evolution (lymphangiosarcoma);
- Disfiguration due to the enlarged limb.

Many patients are young women, and cosmetic considerations have to be included, but this is rarely the only indication for surgery which is usually some degree of functional impairment. With *excisional procedures* it is possible to remove some of the skin and subcutaneous tissues with skin grafting. Several variations of these procedures have been described. A reduction in the size of the limb may be achieved but no procedure is really satisfactory as extensive scarring, sensory loss, and some degree of swelling is usually observed.

Direct procedures try to increase lymph flow and drainage by correcting lymphatic obstruction. Some procedures tend to transfer normal lymphatic channels from a normal area to a lymphoedematous one. In the Thompson procedure longitudinal flaps of dermis are folded beneath the muscles along the medial and the lateral side of the limbs to produce new lymphatic connections between the altered superficial dermal lymphatic system and a normal deep lymphatic system. Results may be good but the presence of new lymphatics has never been shown. Omental flaps have also been used but they have been less successful. With the enteromesenteric bridge method new lymphatic connections have been shown between inguinal lymph nodes and the bowel with long term satisfactory results in a small number of patients. However, these methods require extensive dissection and must be used only in selected patients.

With microvascular surgery new surgical techniques are available.

Lymphovenous anastomosis (Figure 8.5) has been used but prospective studies analyzing results obtained with these methods are not available.

Lymphatic auto-transplant has also been experimented with in a limited number of patients. Lymphatic tissue (nodes) is implanted after being harvested from the healthy limb and fragmented into the affected limb. It has been suggested that this implanted tisue may grow and produce new lymphatic channels in limbs with lymphoedema.

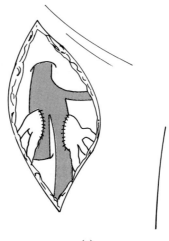

(a)

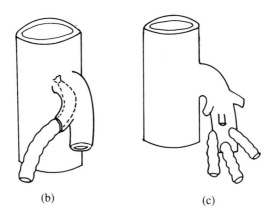

(b)   (c)

Figure 8.5. (a) An example of lympho-venous anastomosis at the sapheno-femoral junction. (b) Lympho-venous intubation according to Cockett. (c) Multiple anastomoses at the sapheno-femoral junction.

Prognosis

If untreated, lymphoedema progresses, producing increasing levels of disability and disfiguration. The enlarged, heavy extremity becomes unusable and infection may recur often. A careful oedema control program must be planned together with the patient and according to her/his lifestyle and social needs. A combination of physical exercise and compression is the key to treatment and control of the evolution of lymphoedema. Cellulitis must be scrupulously avoided and treated aggressively if it does occur. Most patients have real benefits from a severe therapeutic programme. Experience to date with surgery does not clearly indicate the benefits of each procedure, and prospective studies are needed.

CHAPTER 9

DEEP VENOUS THROMBOSIS

Diagnosis

- Swelling, pain, erythema, warmth, discomfort, calf tenderness, positive Homans sign, fever, tachycardia.
- Clinical manifestations may be absent in many patients. Pulmonary embolism may occur without signs or symptoms in the limb.

Introduction

In the USA some 600 000 patients are treated in hospital for deep venous thrombosis (DVT) each year. DVT and pulmonary embolism (PE) are common and sometimes fatal complications of major surgical procedures, particularly those followed by immobilization.

Three major factors have been indicated by Virchow (1856) as the most important initial causes of venous thrombosis:

(1) Vein wall abnormalities (i.e. inflammation, trauma);
(2) Blood flow alterations (stasis);
(3) Alterations in the blood (hypercoagulability) (Table 9.1).

Although may factors are still unclear, thrombosis may be considered a response to even minor injury to the venous structure.

The chain of events producing venous thombosis is summarized in Figure 9.1. Venous thrombi are composed mainly of erythrocytes in a fibrin mesh with few platelets and are therefore defined as *red thrombi*. On the contrary, arterial thrombi are made up of platelet aggregates trapped in fibrin with a few red cells, and are therfore called *white thrombi*. This implies different mechanisms of formation. The precise cause of venous thrombosis is often difficult to define. The thombus formation usually begins in the venous sinuses in the muscles of the legs and in the valve cusps where venous flow is slow or there is some temporary stasis. In these areas an accumulation of activated clotting factors may occur. Platelets are important in the early phases of thrombus formation triggering the coagulation process. As the platelet aggregate grows, it creates turbulent flow augmenting platelet aggregation and release of procoagulants. The venous lumen becomes more compromised, increasing local stasis, which further contributes to the development of the thrombus.

Table 9.1. Situations and clinical problems increasing the risk of venous thrombosis.

Vein wall alterations
Previous history of thrombosis
Inflammation/infection around veins
Venous lesions (cannulation or surgical lesion)
Varicose veins

Stasis
All conditions associated with hypomobility
Impairment in limb mobility
Congestive heart failure
Extrinsic compression of vein by masses (tumours, abscesses, etc.)
External compression (improperly placed bandages, pillows, etc.)
Decreased arterial flow as in shock

Hypercoagulability
Activated protein C resistance
Antithrombin III, protein S and protein C deficiency
Surgery, trauma, injury
Childbirth
Hyperviscosity as in polycytaemia
Neoplastic diseases
Use of oral contraceptives

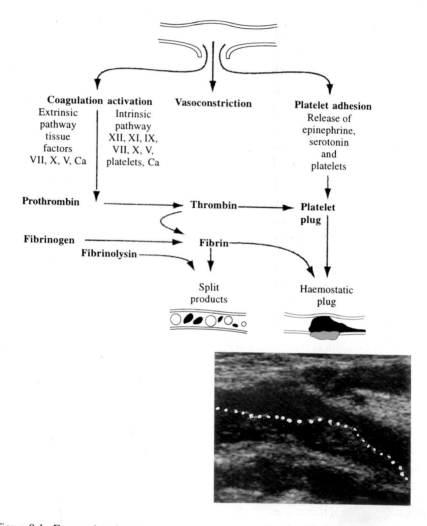

Figure 9.1. Factors involved in the haemostatic process. A popliteal thrombus is shown (b-mode ultrasound). A more echogenic (possibly 2–3 weeks old) part of the thrombus is shown below the dotted line. The echolucent part of the thrombus (above the dotted line) is not visible by ultrasound (same density of blood) but is revealed by the impossibility of compressing the vein under the probe.

Symptoms and Signs

The most important clinical problem in DVT is to establish quickly and objectively that thrombosis has occurred and that the patient needs secondary prophylaxis or treatment (either anticoagulation to avoid the extension of the thrombus and pulmonary embolism or other treatments such as thrombolysis or surgery). The clinical presentation of DVT varies from no signs/symptoms to severe obstruction, pain and systemic signs of inflammation. Most patients complain of pain and discomfort in the involved calf or thigh. The pain may be aggravated by exercise. Depending on the degree of obstruction, limb swelling is variable (from absent to severe). Pulmonary embolism may be associated with dyspnea, chest pain, anxiety tachycardia and fever.

The location of the thrombus determines physical findings. Three major sites of DVT of the lower limbs can be considered (Figure 9.2):

(1) *Localized thrombosis of the calf* may be localized at the sinuses of the soleus muscle veins and the posterior tibial and peroneal veins (Figure 9.3). Calf pain and tenderness may be present while swelling is usually distal or may be slight or even absent (when there is no obstruction).

(2) *Femoral vein thrombosis* is often associated with calf thrombosis. It is associated with pain and tenderness in the distal thigh and popliteal region. Swelling is more prominent than with calf vein thrombosis alone and extends to the level of the knee.

(3) *Iliofemoral venous thrombosis* produces the most severe manifestations, often with massive swelling, pain and tenderness of the entire lower extremity.

Phlegmasia caerulea dolens (meaning painful, swollen blue leg) is a severe form of iliofemoral thrombosis that causes such marked obstruction of venous outflow that cyanosis develops. It can progress to *venous gangrene. Phlegmasia alba dolens* (meaning painful, swollen white leg) is a variant characterized by arterial spasm or compression due to massive oedema resulting in a pale, cool leg with diminished or abolished pulses.

Clinical signs are often unreliable in the diagnosis of DVT. Occasionally tenderness to palpation along any of the involved veins may be observed. With DVT in the calf, active dorsiflexion of the foot often produces calf pain

(Homan's sign), but this sign is unreliable. Tenderness of the calf when the muscles are compressed against the tibia may be a manifestation of inflammation of the deep veins and therefore thrombosis. This finding is also quite unreliable but may be the first clue to DVT.

Differences in the circumference of the affected extremity compared to the unaffected one are often detectable and should be confirmed by measuring. Swelling is one of the most reliable diagnostic signs indicating some degree

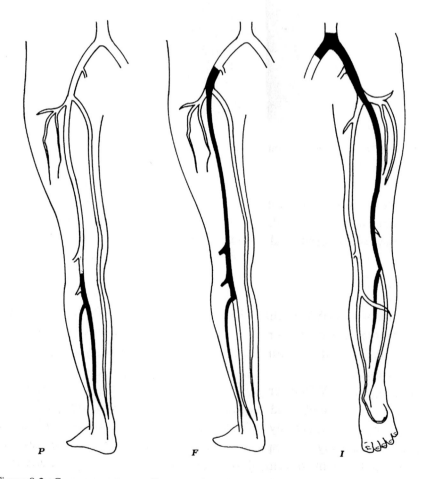

Figure 9.2. Common patterns of venous thrombosis associated with difference in signs and symptoms. P = popliteal thrombosis; F = femoral thrombosis; I = iliac thrombosis.

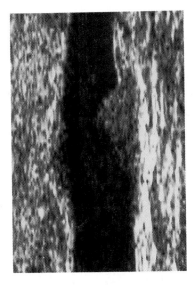

Figure 9.3. Initial formation of a venous thrombus at a valvular cusp.

of obstruction. When collateral venous flow develops, the superficial veins are sometimes visibly dilated, and if the inflammatory component is significant, there may be increased local warmth and erythema.

Diagnostic Tests

The diagnosis of DVT by clinical examination is unreliable, as most patients with thrombosis have few or no signs or symptoms. An objective diagnostic test should be used to confirm the presence of thrombosis and the need for anticoagulation.

Ultrasound. CW Doppler ultrasound is a simple and fast test to search for large occlusive thrombi, and in symptomatic patients it is accurate more than 95% of the time (sensitivity). The test is relatively inexpensive and can be repeated frequently. A simple CW pocket Doppler can indicate stasis or obstructed flow in major veins showing patency or obstruction. In iliofemoral thrombosis the normal respiratory fluctuations in venous flow are stopped. Compression of the calf or thigh while listening for augmented flow in the femoral and popliteal vein is useful for studying the major veins, and iliac, femoral and popliteal veins can be easily evaluated. However, nonocclusive DVT may not be detected with Doppler and false negative results may occur when a thrombus partially obstructs the vein or when extensive collateral venous flow is present. *CW Doppler cannot be used as a reliable screening method to detect limited or initial calf vein thrombosis, and cannot be used to detect limited or initial calf thrombosis or any DVT not associated with some degree of obstruction. Therefore it should not be considered as a valid diagnostic method but only as a screening technique or adjunct to diagnosis.*

By *B-mode ultrasound* the incompressibility of veins under pressure with the probe, the presence of a visible thrombus (echogenicity), and the lack of venous distension with Valsalva's manoeuvre (indicating iliac or femoral thrombosis) are reliable criteria for diagnosing thrombosis. B-mode demonstration of femoral or popliteal vein thrombosis indicates the need for anticoagulation. Localized iliac vein thrombosis may not be detected by B-mode imaging alone but should be diagnosed by color Doppler flow imaging.

Duplex and colour duplex ultrasound combines B-mode imaging with Doppler flow imaging. Colour flow visualizes flow direction or turbulence and flow variations with compression and respiration. Duplex and colour duplex are very accurate in detecting major axial DVT (sensitivity and specificity rates are 90–100%).

With colour duplex after scanning the femoral veins in the supine position and the popliteal vein on standing (weight on the opposite limb) and then scanning all the remaining main superficial and deep veins of both legs in a sitting position requires about 20 minutes. By the use of an abdominal (3.5 MHz) probe the iliac veins and the inferior vena cava can be scanned in the supine position in most patients, obtaining results comparable to phlebography.

Particularly with colour duplex, the flow around the thrombus on compression of the calf allows a very clear and rapid visualization of thrombosis, demonstrating floating thrombi which may cause embolism.

The demonstration of a DVT of the upper limb or subclavian veins and those draining into the superior vena cava is more difficult and less precise.

Ascending phlebography. The test is done with the patient standing and with the weight on the opposite extremity. The contrast medium is injected into a vein on the dorsum of the foot. Calf, popliteal, femoral and iliac veins are visualized. Thrombosis is indicated by:

- Constant filling defects;
- Diversion of flow;
- Abrupt termination of the contrast column;
- Nonfilling of the entire deep venous system or segments.

The sinuses and small veins of the calf muscles are difficult to visualize and the deep femoral vein is opacified in only 50% of patients. However, phlebography demonstrating over 90% of thrombi is considered the most accurate method of investigating DVT. A negative venogram generally excludes the presence of DVT of the lower extremities. It is expensive and impractical to repeat phlebography at frequent intervals. Occasionally a venogram may cause thrombosis.

Venography performed using radioisotopes (*radionuclide venography*) is simple and reliable in detecting major vein occlusion. Both contrast and radionuclide venography are generally performed on an out-patient basis.

Venography is not required when the diagnosis has been established by B-mode or colour duplex. The most important problem in these patients is to decide what type of treatment (i.e. anticoagulation) must be used.

Plethysmography. Plethysmography measures changes in venous flow volume and its changes due to venous outflow obstruction. However, all methods of detecting venous obstruction, such as strain gauge or impedance plethysmography, may be negative in the case of proximal thrombosis associated with good collateral circulation.

Air plethysmography has recently been used to diagnose DVT and to quantify venous obstruction, with good results.

Impedance plethysmography calculates the volume of blood in the limb, measuring changes in electrical resistance. This method can detect iliac, femoral and popliteal obstruction due to thrombosis. The positive predictive value is at least 95% in patients with major DVT producing obstruction. However, impedance plethysmography is not accurate in evaluating calf thrombosis and is insensitive to partially occluding thrombi. This method has been replaced in many vascular centres by ultrasound-based tests. This test is still widely used in the USA, but its use in Europe is limited. Serial screening with ultrasound or IPG is useful for detecting distal or nonocclusive thrombi that may progress to become more clinically significant (i.e. a risk of PE).

Radioactive fibrinogen (RF) test. Circulating fibrinogen becomes incorporated into growing thrombi. If fibrinogen is labelled with a radioactive material (125I), thrombosis can be detected by external scanning over the veins. Its diagnostic applications are limited, as it requires between 12 and 24 hours to complete. Screening with RF indicates that DVT may occur in some 10–30% of general surgical patients and in 50% of orthopaedic or neurosurgical patients. By the RF test it has been shown that DVT often begins during surgery. Signs and symptoms of thrombosis are actually present in only 5–10% of these subjects.

About 90% of postoperative thrombi detected by the RF test are limited (localized to the calf) and probably not dangerous. Some 20% of these localized calf thrombi may progress to the larger veins (popliteal or femoral), causing signs and being a potential source of emboli. The RF test is senstive enough to detect small, localized soleal, tibial and peroneal DVT.

The RF test is considered the most sensitive test for lower limb DVT and the best screening method. However, it does not detect thrombi that are not actively incorporating fibrinogen and it cannot detect femoral, iliac or pelvic thromboses. This test correlates very well with venography, false positive or false negative results are uncommon, and it can be easily repeated after a single dose of RF to follow up the evolution of the thrombi.

The RF test requires the use of nonvirally inactivated blood products, and this has also limited its use.

Blood tests have been developed to detect intravascular coagulation in DVT including measurement of fibrinopeptide A, circulating fibrin monomer complexes, and serum fibrin degradation products (D-dimer). Measurement of the degradation product fragment E is a sensitive test, but the method is complex and not used for practical clinical diagnosis. A negative D-dimer test can be used to rule out the presence of venous thromboembolism (high negative predictive value). However, all blood tests are nonspecific and generally they are not very useful for diagnosis and at this stage they are mainly used for research.

Monoclonal antibody-labelled platelets and fibrin can be used to localize thrombi. It is possible that these methods will allow localization of thrombi not only in the limbs but also elsewhere in the body (e.g. cerebral thrombosis).

Other tests. DVT may be due to an abdominal tumour compressing the iliac veins or the inferior vena cava. Causes of venous compression, such as intra-abdominal masses, should always be considered, particularly in elder patients. Abdominal ultrasound scans, MRI or CT scans are useful for demonstrating extrinsic compression and should be used when needed to evaluate surgical conditions before initiating anticoagulant and fibrinolytic treatment.

Differential diagnosis. The clinical presentation of venous thrombosis is highly variable and often signs and symptoms are mild or absent.

Compression of the popliteal vein by a synovial cyst (Baker's cyst) may mimic a popliteal thrombosis. Acute synovial rupture and extravasation of synovial fluid into the calf muscles may also mimic acute thrombosis (*pseudothrombophlebitis syndrome*). Such patients may have arthropathy of the knee with an effusion and a popliteal mass may be palpable. Ultrasound and arthrography are very useful for establishing the diagnosis.

Contusion of a calf muscle and rupture of the tendon of the plantaris muscle can produce a swollen, painful calf and may be difficult to differentiate from deep venous occlusion. Acute onset of symptoms during exercise and ecchymosis in the calf indicate muscle injury. Ultrasound (indicating a compressible popliteal vein) and (in some patients) phlebography may be required.

Swelling of a limb may be caused by lymphatic or systemic problems. Bilateral swelling of the legs is sometimes seen in bilateral iliac or caval venous thrombosis, but it is more usually of cardiac or renal origin. When *cellulitis* is present, swelling may be acute and associated with inflammation pain and often a wound may be found. Occasionally it is difficult to distinguish an arterial from a venous occlusion. Usually arterial occlusion is associated with pain, there is no swelling, the superficial and veins are not distended while in venous thrombosis, and the superficial veins are full and dilated. Also, sensation in the distal leg disappears soon in acute arterial occlusion while it is still present in thrombosis. In this case a simple pocket Doppler may rapidly establish the correct diagnosis.

Duplex and colour duplex scanning are very effective in differentiating venous thrombosis from other vascular problems. Very occasionally venography is required. The great advantage of duplex and colour duplex is that the test may be repeated after 24–48 hours in case there is any doubt. If serial testing remains negative, anticoagulation and hospital admission for thrombosis may be avoided.

Treatment

The aims of treatment are to prevent the progression of thrombosis with formation of additional or new thrombi, to prevent embolization and to avoid possible venous valve damage.

Physical Measures

Bed rest and leg elevation. It takes some 7–8 days for thrombi to become more adherent to vein walls, and therefore it is common practice to advice bed rest for several days after the onset of signs/symptoms. The patient is confined to bed with the feet elevated 10–20° above heart level. This measure appears to reduce oedema and pain and the increased venous flow reduces the possibilities of formation of new thrombi. However, the need for bed rest is now questioned as reduced mobility may decrease spontaneous fibrinolysis and increase the risk of new thrombosis. Elastic compression of the limb is indicated, because it reduces venous blood pooling and increases the venous flow velocity. Bed rest should be continued until swelling, pain and tenderness have been reduced. Ambulation with elastic (graduated compression stockings) is then permitted. Elastic support and limitations on sitting and standing are generally continued until recanalization and collateral veins start developing.

Drug treatment. Unless there are specific contraindications, anticoagulants should be initiated as soon as possible in every thrombosis at risk of pulmonary embolism. The aims of anticoagulation are:

(1) To prevent the growth of the thrombus;
(2) To avoid the formation of new thrombi;
(3) To prevent pulmonary embolization (PE).

With anticoagulation the dissolution of the thrombus is faster as endogenous fibrinolysis operates unopposed.

Heparin. Heparin therapy should be started as soon as the diagnosis of DVT has been confirmed. Heparin inhibits thrombus formation by neutralizing thrombin and by inhibiting the platelet release reaction. It is of proven benefit in the treatment of DVT and in the prevention of PE. It is not absorbed from the gastrointestinal tract, so it must be given either intravenously or subcutaneously, but the intravenous method is more effective. Intramuscular injection of heparin should be avoided, as it may cause local haemorrhage at the injection site. Bleeding complications are limited if dosage is regulated according to one of the coagulation tests, such as the activated partial thromboplastin time (APTT). Bleeding complications are least if the heparin is given by continuous intravenous infusion. Recurrent episodes of thrombosis and embolism are minimized by administering sufficient heparin by the continuous intravenous route to maintain the APTT at least at 1.5 times control. The amount of heparin required may vary from day to day, so the degree of anticoagulation must be monitored daily. An initial dose of 100 units/kg body weight should be given intravenously and subsequent doses determined by laboratory tests. The anticoagulant effect of *intravenous heparin* is immediate. Most patients initially require 1000–2000 heparin units per hour to achieve adequate anticoagulation.

In the past heparin was generally administered for 7–10 days, the time required for thrombi to become adherent to the vein walls. However, a 5-day treatment with heparin has been shown to be as effective in randomized, prospective studies.

Warfarin therapy should be started with intravenous heparin unless the patient is clinically unstable (for example, he may require thrombolysis or other urgent interventions). If after 5–10 days signs and symptoms (pain, tenderness, etc.) are still present or repeated ultrasound tests indicate growth or extension of the thrombus heparin, treatment may be continued for a longer period. Even with effective heparin treatment the incidence of PE may be some 5%.

Complications. Bleeding is the most important complication of heparin treatment and may be less with *low molecular weight heparins (LMWH)* than with unfractionated heparin. It occurs in 5–10% of patients, particularly in surgical patients with recent surgical wounds or in the gastrointestinal or genitourinary tract. Bleeding may be an important sign of an undiagnosed neoplastic or ulcerated lesion. Protamine sulphate, a heparin inhibitor, is given when bleeding is significant.

Antiplatelet drugs interfering with platelet aggregation in heparinized patients may interfere with primary haemostasis and coagulation. Platelet counts should be obtained before and during heparin therapy as *thrombocytopaenia* (due to a heparin-induced antiplatelet antibody) may occur with heparin treatment. Thrombocytopaenia usually occurs 5–7 days after heparin is started; it may be persistent and severe and sometimes is associated with haemorrhage, recurrent thrombosis or embolism.

The treatment with LMWH is associated with less bleeding complications. As with LMWH, laboratory monitoring is not needed; it is possible to treat DVT directly at home.

Oral anticoagulants. Coumarin derivatives block the biological activity of four vitamin-K-dependent clotting factors (*prothrombin and factors VII, IX and X*). The anticoagulant effects are delayed until the biologically active factors (gamma carboxylated) are cleared from the blood; therefore the onset of action of oral anticoagulants is slow. Treatment reduces the prothrombin time and is used for long term prophylaxis or treatment after discontinuing heparin. As oral anticoagulants inhibit the synthesis of the anticoagulant proteins C and S and protein C has a very short half-life, there is a period of relative hypercoagulability during the first days of treatment with the oral anticoagulant. Therefore warfarin should be started during the first or second day of heparin treatment, discontinuing heparin only after the prothrombin time has been at therapeutic levels for a few days. The therapeutic range for oral anticoagulants has been established by prospecive clinical trials. The dose increasing the prothrombin time to 2–2.5 the normal value is known to be excessive as an equal antithrombotic effect can be achieved with a prothrombin time of 1.35–1.6 times the control value. Many laboratories report together with prothrombin time the *International Normalized Ratio (INR)*. The INR considers variations in reactivity of reagents used to determine prothrombin time.

Using the INR the recommended anticoagulant intensity for treating DVT is an INR of 2–3.

After DVT, oral anticoagulation should be continued for at least three months since this is the time required for development of venous collaterals and also the time during which most recurrences of thrombosis occur.

After submassive PE or iliac-femoral DVT , six months of anticoagulation is usually indicated. Interaction between oral anticoagulants and and many other drugs (e.g. H_2 receptor blockers, nonsteroidal anti-inflammatory agents, some antibiotics,barbiturates) may increase the possibility of complications, and therefore patients on oral anticoagulants must be cautioned againts the use of any drugs without prior discussion with their physician.

Bleeding complications occur in 5–10% of patients. Excessive prolongation of the prothrombin time can be treated with vitamin K. Self-administered, low dose heparin therapy is also used as an alternative to warfarin in the long term management of thromboembolic disorders and appears to be associated with fewer bleeding complications than heparin therapy.

Recurrent thromboembolism occurs in less than 2% of effectively treated patients. Where DVT appears to have occurred spontaneously consideration should be given to a thrombophilia screening which may indicate the need for permanent anticoagulation.

Thrombolysis

Fibrinolytic activators (streptokinase and urokinase and tissue plasminogen activator (t-PA)) produce lysis of fresh thrombi. These drugs produce rapid clearance of the occluded veins and may preserve competency and function of venous valves better than heparin treatment. Lytic therapy may be an effective method for preventing the post-thrombotic syndrome and normal venous function may be preserved in about 40% of patients after fibrinolytic therapy if given early enough. This treatment has no advantages over heparin when DVT had been present for more than 72 hours and in the prevention of recurrent DVT. Particularly in surgical patients, bleeding is more common than with conventional anticoagulants. These drugs are very expensive.

Both systemic infusion and catheter-directed thrombolysis have been used with success.

t-PA is more thrombin-specific and its action is more rapid than other fibrinolytic agents. Thrombolysis of ileofemoral DVT may case proximal embolisation and it is usually combined with the placement of a temporary vena caval filter.

Ancrod (Arvin) reduces plasma fibrinogen by cleavage of fibrinopeptide A. This drug produces intravascular defibrination. It is effective for DVT but does not appear to be superior to heparin. This drug has been effectively used in patients who develop heparin-induced thrombocytopaenia and who require ongoing anticoagulation. Bleeding complications are treated with the Arvin antidote (which may cause anaphylaxis), freeze-dried fibrinogen, or if this is not available, fresh plasma.

Complications of DVT. The most important *acute complications* are PE and acute, severe obstruction leading to venous gangrene. *Chronic complications* are chronic venous insufficiency and the postphlebitic syndrome, which may lead to ulcerations and secondary varicosity. The *objectives of treatment* of acute DVT are to prevent PE, one of the major killers in the hospital, further swelling of the limb and the post-thrombotic syndrome.

The following points must be remembered:

(1) The risk of mortality from PE increases with the proximity of the thrombus. VQ scans have demonstrated PE in about 30% in calf thrombosis, in about 50% in iliofemoral thrombosis and in about 65% in thrombosis extending to the inferior vena cava.

(2) Further swelling of the leg may lead to an acute compartment syndrome with *phlegmasia caerulea dolens, venous gangrene* and loss of the limb. This is a rare condition which requires immediate surgical intervention with fasciotomy and/or thrombectomy or thrombolysis.

(3) The post-thrombotic syndrome may lead to chronic venous insufficiency with swelling of the leg, hyperpigmentation, skin induration, venous claudication and ulcerations.

Surgical treatment of venous thrombosis. The majority of patients with DVT are managed by anticoagulation. Lysis of the thrombus depends on endogenous thrombolysis, which requires weeks to months for recanalization. This may lead to destruction of the valves present within the affected segment. Therefore anticoagulation may be of limited value in preventing the post-thrombotic syndrome which usually follows the loss of venous valve function.

Thrombolytic therapy seems a logical approach to the problem but more prospective clinical trials are required to prove its value over conservative management or surgery.

In acute iliofemoral thrombosis, *surgical thrombectomy* (often combined with a temporary arteriovenous fistula) may be considered. There are indications for surgery if the history of swelling of the thigh indicates that iliac obstruction is less that a week old and the life expectancy of the patient is more than 10 years.

The objectives of surgery are to prevent fatal PE, further swelling of the leg with development of phlegmasia caerulea dolens and venous gangrene, and evolution to the post-thrombotic syndrome.

Several studies indicate no mortality from peroperative PE and no difference in nonfatal PE compared with control groups treated with anticoagulation alone. Surgery has an immediate positive effect on swelling of the leg and it is clearly indicated if phlegmasia caerulea dolens has already developed. Thrombectomy has showed a significant improvement of iliac vein patency and valvular funtion and should thereby prevent the development of the post-thrombotic syndrome.

Venous interruption. The rationale of venous interruption is the prevention of recurrent and potentially fatal PE by trapping emboli in peripheral venous segments. In patients with a single pulmonary embolus treated effectively with anticoagulants, fatal PE is rare (1–2%). Surgery is indicated for the patient who fails to respond to anticoagulants or with specific contraindications to its use or thrombectomy. Ligation of the superficial femoral vein prevents embolization from distal muscular and deep veins and, rarely, is followed by chronic venous disfunction. However, this procedure does not stop embolization from more proximal venous segments. As most fatal pulmonary emboli arise from iliac or pelvic veins, venous interruption in the extremities has been replaced by techniques that trap emboli in the inferior vena cava (IVC) (Figure 9.4). Since caval ligation was introduced by Homans in 1944, numerous methods have been developed and applied clinically. The need to preserve flow in the IVC and to preserve a normal distal venous pressure stimulated the development of caval plication techniques using sutures or serrated clips. The Adams–De-Weese clips are still used as a surgical approach to IVC thrombosis. Early transvenous devices were susceptible to proximal

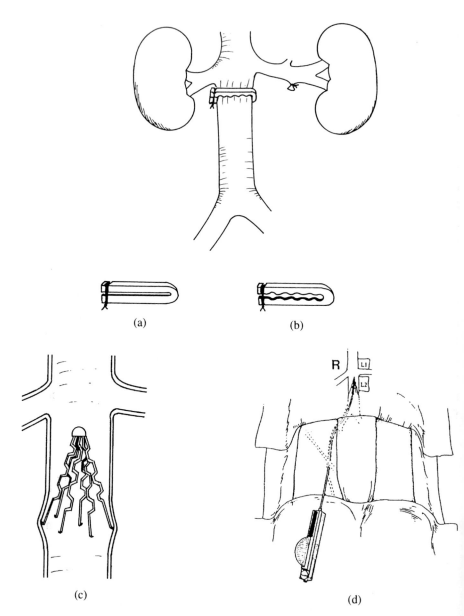

(a)

(b)

(c)

(d)

Figure 9.4. Prevention of PE with partial interruption of the vena cava to trap large emboli. The Moretz caval clip (left) and the Miles teflon clip (right) are among the most used. They are usually placed just distally to the renal veins. The gonadal veins should be ligated. The Greenfield intracaval filter (c) may be inserted transcutaneously (d).

migration or produced unacceptable morbidity from occlusion of the IVC. There are now devices small enough to be safely introduced percutaneoulsy. To be effective an IVC filter must filter emboli, maintain IVC patency and remain in position. The *indications* for insertion of a caval filter vary widely around the world. In patients with objective documentation of DVT and PE these are our indications:

(1) Contraindication to anticoagulation;
(2) Failure of anticoagulation (i.e. PE on adequate treatment);
(3) Complications of anticoagulation;
(4) Prophylaxis in high risk patients with DVT;
(5) Following pulmonary embolectomy.
(6) Prior to abdominal surgery.
(7) Temporary filter during thrombolysis.

Comparison of different filters is difficult since randomized prospective studies are not available and studies of individual filters differ in follow-up method, placement of indications and patient population. The current standard for implantable vena cava devices is the stainless steel Greenfield filter. It has above 90% efficiency in preventing recurrent PE and the same high patency rate. Other filters currently available are the nitinol filter, the Gunther filter, the bird's nest filter, the Venatech filter and, recently, the titanium Greenfield filter.

CHAPTER 10

PULMONARY THROMBOEMBOLISM

Diagnosis

- History and clinical findings of DVT are often absent.
- PE occurs most commonly in very sick, elderly, immobilized or traumatized patients.
- Large pulmonary emboli cause sudden onset of dyspnoea, and anxiety. Chest pain may be present and signs of acute right heart failure and circulatory collapse may follow promptly.
- Pulmonary infarction is characterized by cough, haemoptysis, less severe dyspnoea, pleuritic pain and peripheral x-ray density in the lung.
- The diagnosis is suggested by a ventilation perfusion lung scan but established only by a pulmonary angiogram.

Introduction and General Considerations

It is estimated that in the USA fatal PE (more than 600 000 cases) is the third most frequent cause of death (after myocardial infarction and stroke), responsible for at least 5% of postoperative deaths (some 200 000 deaths/ year). Nonfatal attacks are 3–5 times more frequent than fatal PE. About one-fourth to one-half of cases of fatal PE occur in patients with an otherwise good prognosis. Pulmonary thromboembolism is therefore relatively common and may occur in almost any clinical setting. However, PE is rarely observed in healthy young patients while elderly, immobilized, sick or traumatized patients have the highest incidence. The incidence of PE is proportional to the age of the patient and the duration of the illness. Heart disease appears to be the major risk factor. A higher risk of PE is also present during pregnancy and the puerperium. Cardiac failure, surgical procedures and oral contraceptive use are other factors affecting the incidence of PE. DVT of the legs, which may be demonstrated only in some 30–40% of patients with PE, is the most common cause of embolization. Immobilization in bed, reduced mobility and exercise may double the incidence of PE. Iliac and femoral veins are the source of most pulmonary emboli, but emboli can also originate in other systemic veins, such as in perineal and axillary-subclavian DVT. Thrombosis of smaller veins (i.e. in the calf) rarely causes severe PE. Only thrombi produced in veins the size of the iliac and femoral veins are large enough to produce emboli with major clinical sequelae. PE may be also caused by *tumour embolization of the lungs* (i.e. renal cell carcinoma). *Cardiac tumours* arising in the right atrium and right ventricle may also cause extensive PE. In most patients PE involves lobar arteries in each lung. As the occlusion of a pulmonary artery affects respiration, the global pulmonary circulation, the heart and the bronchial circulation, several different mechanisms are involved in the responses to PE. Reflex changes are probably secondary to microembolization and may cause tachypnoea, pulmonary hypertension and systemic hypotension. Vasoactive amines arising from the emboli and prostaglandins are possibly involved in the response to PE.

PE increases pulmonary arterial resistance and pulmonary arterial pressure, increasing also right ventricular work. Signs and symptoms are both related to the extent of arterial obstruction and to the pre-embolic situations of the cardiovascular system. The degree of cardiovascular impairment is proportional to the extent of the arterial obstruction when there are no pre-existing cardiopulmonary problems. When the cardiorespiratory system is chronically impaired, even limited PE may be fatal or cause severe signs and symptoms.

Diagnosis

Signs and symptoms of PE may be similar to those of other cardiorespiratory diseases. Dyspnoea and tachypnoea are frequent clinical observations. Haemoptysis (present in about 20% of patients) in association with pleural friction rub (8–10%), gallop rhythm, cyanosis (10% of patients) and chest splinting are present together in only 15% of patients. Clinical symptoms and signs of DVT are present in about one-third of patients, but when noninvasive investigations are used the percentage of patients with documented DVT may increase to some 45%. Dyspnoea is often present (two-thirds of patients), often associated with chest pain (60% of patients). Tachycardia is present in 60%, and altered mental status is observed in some 25% of patients. Accentuation of the pulmonary second sound is common. The triad *dyspnoea + chest pain + haemoptysis* is usually present only in 15% of patients. Bronchoconstriction is often present. Chest pain is frequent with massive PE but rarely observed with small emboli and often described as a deep, substernal tightness. In the case of severe right ventricular disfunction a wide, almost fixed splitting of the second heart sound is a very severe prognostic sign. A friction rub may be heard over the lung bases, because the lower lobes are the most frequent location of PE. Tachypnoea and tachycardia are the most common findings. Marked tachycardia and tachypnoea indicate massive PE. An increase in temperature is commonly observed.

Laboratory Findings

Arterial blood gas analysis may be useful. Hypoxaemia is nonspecific and may be transient. When arterial hypoxaemia is not present PE is unlikely.

Imaging Studies

A *chest x-ray* may be normal (there is no diagnostic radiologic sign of PE on the plain chest film). With massive PE, there is usually no evidence of congestion. The peripheral lung fields are blanched because of diminished blood flow. Typical wedge-shaped peripheral infiltrates may appear later. A pleural effusion may also be present. A reliable diagnossis depends on pulmonary angiography or a radioisotope perfusion scan.

A *pulmonary radioisotope perfusion scan* (Figure 10.1) is performed by the intravenous injection of serum albumin labelled with technetium (^{99m}Tc) or ^{131}I and injected intravenously. This method demonstrates the distribution of pulmonary arterial flow, revealing areas of decreased perfusion. The pulmonary perfusion scan is useful in confirming signs and symptoms of PE before treatment is started. It can be repeated with minimal discomfort to the patient and is the best means of following the evolution of PE. Lesions present

RPO   **POST**   **LPO**

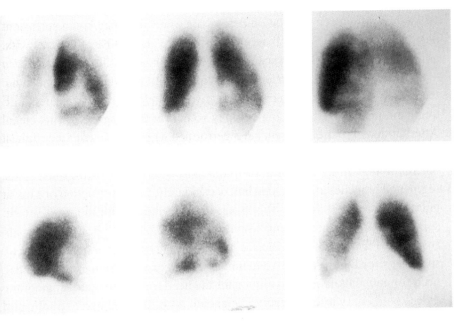

L.L.   **ANT**   **R.L.**

Figure 10.1. A pulmonary radioisotope perfusion scan is performed by intravenous injection of serum albumin labelled with technetium (^{99m}Tc) or ^{131}I and injected intravenously. This method demonstrates the distribution of pulmonary arterial flow, revealing areas of decreased perfusion.

on the plain chest film, such as pneumonitis, atelectasis, emphysematous bullae, or neoplasm, demonstrate a defect on scan (false-positive scan). Such abnormal areas must be excluded from consideration by a simultaneous plain chest x-ray or ventilation scan (or both). High probability perfusion scans are very specific for PE and correlate well with angiography. Normal or near normal perfusion scans exclude significant PE. All other lung scan abnormalities are nondiagnostic and further studies are required to establish a diagnosis.

^{133}*Xenon ventilation scanning* increases the sensitivity of perfusion scans, because it differentiates underperfused and underventilated areas. The scan indicates the distribution of the inhaled gas, facilitating the interpretation of perfusion scans. Typically PE causes perfusion defects in an area of normal ventilation. However, ventilation defects are often associated with perfusion defects in submassive embolism. PE is present in about 90% of patients with a high probability perfusion scan and a ventilation–perfusion mismatch.

Selective pulmonary arteriography is the definitive method for establishing the diagnosis. The seriousness of the disease and the significant risks of treatment justify the use of angiography whenever the diagnosis is not clear. Arteriography is extremely reliable if performed within 48 hours of the clinical episode. The diagnosis is established by demonstration of unequivocal obstruction or filling defects in the pulmonary arterial tree. Most often lobar segmental branches are occluded but, occasionally, total obstruction of a main pulmonary artery is found. This is usually associated with the most severe symptoms. Before proceeding to pulmonary angiography in a patient with suspected PE and a nondiagnostic lung scan pattern, it is recommended to study legs for DVT. A positive noninvasive test or venogram establishes the need for anticoagulation and eliminates the need for a pulmonary angiogram unless pulmonary artery surgery is planned. Also, 2D echocardiography has been shown to be an effective noninvasive test for pulmonary embolism and may eliminate the need for pulmonary angiography. Increased right ventricular pressures and volumes and decreased right ventricular wall motion are indicative of acute PE. These studies can also be used to follow the outcome of thrombolytic therapy.

Electrocardiography. About 15% of patients with PE have acute electrocardiographic changes, the most common abnormalities being T-wave inversion and ST segment depression (resulting from myocardial ischaemia, from decreased cardiac output and arterial pressure, and increased right ventricular pressure). Most often electrocardiographic changes are nonspecific, but the test is useful in diagnosing other conditions that may explain the patient's signs/symptoms.

Differential Diagnosis

Differential diagnosis includes pneumonia, myocardial infarction, congestive heart failure, angina pectoris, atelectasis, lung abscess, tuberculosis, pulmonary neoplasm, viral pleuritis, asthma and pericarditis.

The sudden onset of atrial fibrillation in a patient without pre-existing cardiac disease as well as the sudden worsening of congestive heart failure suggest PE. Acute cardiopulmonary disorders such as myocardial infarction, dissecting aortic aneurysm and pneumothorax may be confused with massive PE; they cause similar signs/symptoms (substernal discomfort, dyspnoea, tachycardia and electrocardiographic changes).

Pulmonary infarction. Pulmonary embolism and infarction are not synonymous, as less than 10% of pulmonary emboli produce infarction. A true pulmonary infarct is seldom produced in a normal lung, and even complete ligation of the pulmonary artery does not lead to infarction. Pulmonary infarcts are usually peripheral and most often in the lower lobes. Infarcts are related to occlusion of a pulmonary artery when severe clinical conditions affecting the lung (i.e. chronic lung disease, infection or congestive heart failure) are already present.

The prevention of PE. The *primary prevention* of DVT and PE is discussed in the following chapter. *Secondary prevention* of PE (i.e. in the case of recurrent embolization in subjects adequately treated with anticoagulation) indicates the need for a caval filter.

Treatment

Medical treatment. The patient's limbs should be elevated to reduce stasis. Graduated compression stockings appear effective in reducing stasis and decreasing the rate of growth of the thrombus. After an *intravenous bolus of heparin* (e.g. 10 000 units), heparin is administered by continuous intravenous infusion for 5–6 days. *Oral anticoagulants* are started at the same time as the heparin infusion unless the patient is clinically unstable. Heparin is discontinued 2–3 days after a one-stage prothrombin time of 1.3–1.5 times the control (INR 2.0–3.0) has been reached. Oral anticoagulants are usually continued for a period of 3–6 months.

Thrombolytic treatment is indicated in patients in shock or right heart failure as well as in patients with severe pulmonary hypertension who may die if additional PE occurs.

The following regimens appear to be equally effective:

Urokinase: 4.400 IU/kg intravenously as an initial dose followed by 4.400 IU/kg/h for 12 hours;

Streptokinase: 250,000 IU intravenously in 30 minutes, followed by 100.000 IU/h for 24 hours;

Alteplase (recombinant tissue plasminogen activator) 90–100 mg intravenously in 7 hours. Heparin is always administered after the thrombolytic infusion is completed.

The most common *complication* of thrombolysis is bleeding occurring at surgical wounds, catheterization sites and sites of recent stroke. Therefore lytic treatment should not be used within three weeks after the surgery, trauma or parturition. Streptokinase is pyrogenic and may cause allergy.

Surgical treatment, performed in cardiopulmonary bypass, is life-saving in selected patients with massive embolism. The principal indication for *pulmonary embolectomy* is severe, refractory hypotension after resuscitation in subjects with massive embolism proved by lung scan or pulmonary arteriogram and who have had no response or have contraindications to thrombolytic therapy. Most patients previously thought to require embolectomy are now treated medically and respond favourably to heparinization, vasopressors and inotropic agents.

In many of these patients more than half of the pulmonary arterial system is occluded, with the exception of patients with pre-existing cardiac or respiratory insufficiency. A survival rate of 75–80% may be obtained.

Surgical treatment or local thrombolysis of the thrombus causing repeated embolization is also used in some selected patients.

Transvenous methods are now used more frequently to remove pulmonary emboli using large suction catheters inserted through a peripheral (i.e femoral) vein. With catheterization, thrombolysis may be directed to the affected pulmonary arteries. Catheter-based methods are much simpler and cost-effective and may directly follow angiography. They are also less stressful and safer to the patient and, whenever possible, are preferable to surgical embolectomy. In these patients the placement of a *caval filter* is carried out at the same time.

Prognosis

Of the more than 600 000 symptomatic episodes of PE, only 10–12% in the USA each year die within 1 hour. If diagnosis is not made, about 30% of undiagnosed/untreated patients die, mostly as the result of recurrent episodes of PE. Most patients survive PE as the embolus is small, the initial pulmonary arterial obstruction is limited and nonlethal, and lysis of emboli is fast. In patients who survive long enough for the diagnosis to be established and adequate therapy to be instituted, death due to PE is relatively uncommon. After PE progressive resolution of obstruction, following lysis and revascularization of the occluded arteries, is usually observed in a few weeks. The emboli are removed by the combined action of macrophages and by local thrombolysis. Partial resolution of pulmonary thromboembolic obstruction can be detected in most patients by lung scanning or arteriography within a few days after the initial episode. The haemodynamic improvement depends on the revascularization of the pulmonary vascular obstruction.

The acute prognosis is generally determined by the presence of associated clinical conditions (mainly cardiac and respiratory insufficiency). Complete resolution of the obstruction is the usual course. Extensive and repeated pulmonary emboli produce chronic respiratory insufficiency, pulmonary hypertension and right ventricular failure (*cor pulmonale*), which is very difficult to treat. In young subjects, appropriately treated, the prognosis of PE is good when the diagnosis and treatment are prompt. In elderly, sick patients the prognosis is more severe and is mainly determined by comcomitant diseases.

CHAPTER 11

PREVENTION OF VENOUS THROMBOEMBOLISM

DVT and PE are major health problems, with potentially serious outcomes. PE may be fatal or lead to a risk for the development of pulmonary hypertension from recurrent embolism and post-thrombotic venous insufficiency. Both have a great impact on health care costs. Epidemiological data indicate the rate of DVT each year to be around 160 per 100 000 in the general population; the rate of fatal PE is 60 and the number of venous ulcers is 200. The proportion of ulceration due to DVT is still unknown.

Attitudes towards prophylaxis show great regional variations. This is true for the definition of risk groups, the proportion of patients receiving prophylaxis and the prophylactic method chosen.

SURGICAL PATIENTS. Patients who sustain major trauma or undergo prolonged operative procedures without anticoagulation are at risk for developing venous thromboembolic disease. The degree of risk is increased by different factors (age, obesity, malignancy, prior history of venous thrombosis, varicose veins, recent operative procedures and thrombophilic states), as seen in Table 11.1. These factors are modified by general care including operative duration (Table 11.2), type of anaesthesia, pre- and postoperative immobility, level of hydration and presence of sepsis.

MEDICAL PATIENTS. There are less data available in medical than in surgical patients. An increased risk of venous thromboembolism has been shown in patients with acute myocardial infarction, cerebrovascular accidents and immobilized general medical patients.

GYNAECOLOGY AND OBSTETRICS. The reported overall incidence of thromboembolic complications in gynaecologic surgery patients is similar to

Table 11.1. Factors increasing the risk of venous thrombosis.

Abnormal vein wall

Varicose veins
Previous DVT
Trauma to vein walls (cannulation)
Inflammatory process around the veins (especially pelvic)

Venous stasis

Bed rest
Prolonged incorrect position (leg dependency)
Restriction of leg motion (cast, paralysis, postoperative pain)
Congestive heart failure
Extrinsic compression of veins (tumours)
External compression (pillows, bandages)
Decreased arterial flow (shock)

Hypercoagulability

Trauma (surgery, childbirth, injury)
Hyperviscosity
Tumours
Hormones, contraceptives
Deficiency of protein C, protein S and antithrombin III

Table 11.2. Risk groups in trauma and surgery in order of decreasing frequency of DVT.

Spinal cord injury	75–80%
Knee arthroplasty	↓
Leg amputation	↓
Hip fracture surgery	↓
Hip arthroplasty	↓
Lower limb fracture	↓
Open prostatectomy	↓
General abdominal surgery	↓
Gynaecological surgery	↓
Kidney transplantation	↓
Noncardiac thoracic surgery	↓
Neurosurgery	↓
Open meniscectomy	20–25%

that observed in general surgery. PE is a leading cause of death following gynaecological cancer surgery. In pregnancy, DVT occurs in 0.13–0.5/1000 in the antepartum period and 0.61–1.5/1000 in postpartum patients. PE is a leading cause of maternal mortality. Risk factors associated with DVT include the factors included in the surgical section. There is an increased risk of venous thrombosis in women taking oral contraceptives containing more than 50 micrograms or more of oestrogen. However, there are only limited data regarding current low dose oral contraceptives and hormone replacement therapy. Other risk factors associated with DVT/PE in pregnancy include Caesarian section, advanced maternal age and thrombophilic states.

PREDISPOSING HAEMATOLOGICAL CAUSES AND INDICATIONS FOR SCREENING. Congenital predisposition to thrombosis (thrombophilia) is rare but should be considered in patients defined as having had a documented unexplained thrombotic episode below the age of 40, recurrent DVT and a positive family history. The frequency of congenital thrombophilia in consecutive patients with confirmed thrombosis is approximately 8%. Activated protein C resistance is the most common inhibitor deficit predisposing one to thrombosis, with as many as 60% of patients with recurrent DVT having this abnormality. The role of activated protein C resistance in the pathogenesis of idiopathic DVT and DVT occurring in pregnancy, cancer and other high risk states will be clarified by the epidemiological studies currently being performed. In addition a number of acquired haematological abnormalities are associated with a predisposition to venous thromboembolism (e.g. lupus anticoagulant, anticardiolipin, myeloproliferative disease).

The recommended screening tests are:

General: complete blood count including platelets.

Congenital: antithrombin III, protein C, protein S.

Acquired: activated partial thromboplastin time (APTT), anticardiolipin antibody.

Plasminogen, plasminogen and prourokinase activator inhibitor activity, tissue plasminogen activator activity, pre- and post-stress lysis may be considered to rule out an abnormality in the fibrinolytic system if the above tests are normal. But the clinical relevance of abnormalities in the fibrinolytic system is uncertain.

Patients with congenital thrombophilia should be considered at high risk for thromboembolism and should receive appropriate prophylaxis according to the clinical setting.

In *symptomatic patients with congenital thrombophilia* the duration of the treatment is unknown and should be considered case by case taking into account the benefit–risk ratio for the individual. In *asymptomatic patients with congenital thrombophilia* the value of primary prophylaxis is not known, but patients should be protected during surgery or during any medical condition associated with an increased risk of thrombosis.

Pregnant women with thrombophilia are a special subgroup and are at risk throughout pregnancy. They should be considered for thromboprophylaxis. The period of risk begins early in the first trimester in pregnancy, particularly in those with antithrombin III deficiency.

In *patients with acquired haematological abnormalities*, the decision regarding primary prophylaxis should be made on an individual basis.

ORAL ESTROGEN CONTRACEPTION AND PREDISPOSITION TO VENOUS THROMBOSIS. There is epidemiological evidence to suggest a relationship between oestrogen containing oral contraceptives and venous thromboembolism. Therefore the oral contraceptive pill is contraindicated in patients with thrombophilia.

SCREENING FOR THROMBOEMBOLISM. Routine screening for asymptomatic pulmonary emboli is neither necessary nor cost-effective. It is well documented that the majority of pulmonary emboli and the majority of fatal PE occur following asymptomatic DVT. Therefore it is important to diagnose both asymptomatic calf and proximal thrombi when studying the incidence of DVT.

In *low and medium risk patients* who are protected by an established prophylactic method, no routine screening for DVT is needed as the screening is not cost-effective in these categories. In *high risk patients*, even with established prophylaxis, the incidence of asymptomatic DVT is significant and screening for DVT may be useful.

Practical methods for DVT screening are B-mode ultrasound and colour duplex scanning. The simple CW Doppler is not reliable for DVT. B-mode ultrasound and colour duplex are preferred to venography, which is expensive and produces more complications.

PROPHYLAXIS IN GENERAL SURGERY AND UROLOGY. Graduated compression stockings have been shown to be effective in reducing the incidence of DVT in young patients (>45), with mild to moderate risk. Intermittent pneumatic compression (IPC) is also effective in reducing the incidence of DVT. There are insufficient data covering other methods of mechanical prophylaxis. There is little evidence that antiplatelet agents are effective in reducing the incidence of thromboembolism and there are insufficient data to support the use of oral anticoagulants for primary thrombobembolism prophylaxis. Dextran has been shown to be effective in reducing fatal PE but has risks of fluid overload and anaphylaxis. Hepten can reduce this risk. There is only weak evidence to suggest that it reduces DVT.

Low dose heparin is effective in reducing both DVT and PE. Low molecular weight heparins (LMWH) also appear to be effective in general surgical patients in reducing the incidence of DVT and PE, and they are more practical (one daily dose). There are insufficient data on the use of heparinoids in general surgery. Combinations of mechanical and pharmacological methods (heparin) may be more effective.

Known *risk factors* allow us to place patients in the categories of low, medium and high risk of developing thromboembolism.

Low risk patients may receive prophylaxis and graduated compression stockings may be considered. The data are insufficient to make this a mandatory requirement. In all *medium risk patients* LMWH or low dose heparins are effective and may be combined with graduated stockings. An alternative recommendation may be IPC used continuously and combined with graduated compression stockings until the patient is ambulant.

All high risk patients should receive prophylaxis. Apart from single modalities that have been shown to be effective and safe, such as low dose heparin and LMWH, pharmacological and mechanical methods may be combined.

Prophylaxis should be initiated preoperatively and continued for 7–10 days. Consideration should be given to extending prophylaxis when the hospital stay is prolonged or the risk continues. For women taking oral contraceptives, if they cannot be stopped 4–6 weeks before surgery, then consideration should be given to increasing the level of prophylaxis. Patients with a high risk of bleeding either from known coagulation disorder or from specific surgical procedures are better treated with mechanical methods of prophylaxis.

NEUROSURGERY. Neurosurgical patients should be considered for mechanical methods of prophylaxis (i.e. graduated stockings and IPC).

ORTHOPAEDIC SURGERY AND TRAUMA. Patients undergoing elective or emergency operations are at high risk of developing postoperative DVT/ PE. Total hip replacement without prophylaxis is associated with a high incidence of DVT (about 50%) and PE, which in 1–3% is fatal. In addition patients are also at risk of developing the late sequelae of DVT (postphlebitic syndrome), the incidence of which is approximately 50% at five years after an episode of DVT. These observations emphasize the need to protect high risk patients by routine prophylaxis.

Methods of prophylaxis which have been used in this group include aspirin, dextran, fixed low dose unfractionated heparin (FLUDH), adjusted dose heparin, addition of dihydroergotamine to FLDUH, fixed minidose and full dose of oral anticoagulant therapy, external pneumatic compression, LMWH and some heparinoids. The following recommendations are made:

ELECTIVE SURGERY. There is insufficient evidence to recommend antiplatelet drugs for prophylaxis. Dextran is only moderately effective and has risks of fluid overload and anaphylaxis. Fixed low dose unfractioned heparin prophylaxis (5000 bid/tid) is moderately effective, but increasing the dosage enhances the bleeding risk. Adjusting the heparin dosage to the results of a coagulation assay is more effective, but difficult to manage. The addition of dihydroegotamine (DHE) to FLDUH enhances effectiveness, but may cause vasospasm. Adjusting the dose of oral anticoagulants to the appropriate INR improves efficacy. IPC with and without graduated stockings is effective but has some practical limitations. Fixed dose LMWH is very effective. Also, some heparinoids have been used for prophylaxis with good results but the amount of data is limited. The dosage, efficacy and safety of each product need to be considered separately. Prophylaxis should be started preoperatively and continued to 7–10 days or until the patients are fully ambulant.

Experience with fixed low dose heparin indicates that there is no evidence that preoperative anticoagulant prophylaxis enhances the risk of haemorrhage associated with spinal or epidural anaesthesia.

A limited number of studies are available in patients undergoing knee replacement. Results do not permit firm recommendations, but the modalities effective in patients undergoing hip replacement can also be applied in this category, with LMWH being the most effective.

EMERGENCY SURGERY. The prophylactic modalities used for hip fracture and other severe fractures should be started as soon as possible and are comparable to those for elective hip surgery. DHE/heparin is contraindicated.

OBSTETRICS AND GYNAECOLOGY

GYNAECOLOGICAL SURGERY. Low risk patients may receive prophylaxis on an individual basis. Graduated stockings should be considered.

Moderate risk patients are treated with low dose heparin (5000 units, bid). IPC might also be considered, since it has been shown to be effective in higher risk patients. Dextran and warfarin are not recommended for routine prophylaxis but may have a role when LDH is contraindicated. LMWH is also effective. Data concerning the use of graduated stockings in moderate risk gynaecological surgery are insufficient. The use of combination oral contraceptives may be associated with increased risk of DVT in patients undergoing gynaecological surgery. Discontinuation of oral contraceptives 4–6 weeks before surgery should be considered. If oral contraceptives have not been discontinued, prophylaxis should be provided in these patients.

In *high risk patients* undergoing gynaecological surgery, low dose heparin (5000 units every 8 hours) or IPC used continuously for at least 5 days provides effective prophylaxis. Prophylaxis with combined methods and for extended periods need to be defined better. LMWH is also used in these patients, with good results. Data evaluating graduated stockings in high risk gynaecological surgery patients are insufficient.

PREGNANCY. Low dose heparin prophylaxis is commonly used in pregnant patients at high risk of DVT and PE, although data from controlled trials are lacking on the efficacy of this prophylaxis. There are also insufficient data on either the optimum timing or the dosing schedule of low dose heparin prophylaxis. Oral anticoagulants are contraindicated in the first trimester (due to embryopathies). Also, they are associated with foetal alterations in the second trimester and increased maternal–foetal bleeding in the second and third trimesters. Therefore oral anticoagulants should not be used during pregnancy. The benefits of prophylaxis have not been clearly demonstrated in Caesarean section in patients who have no additional risk factors. Perioperative and postpartum prophylaxis may be seriously considered in the presence of additional risk factors. There are still limited data on the use of LMWH or mechanical methods in pregnancy. Women who develop DVT and/or PE during pregnancy should be treated with therapeutic levels of heparin. Heparin should be continued throughout the duration of pregnancy, labour and delivery. Anticoagulation is usually continued for at least 4–6 weeks postpartum (the optimal duration of treatment has not been established).

Patients who develop DVT/PE during pregnancy or the puerperium should be referred for haematological screening.

PROPHYLAXIS IN MEDICAL PATIENTS. There is less information available for medical patients than for surgical patients. However, an increased risk of venous thromboembolism has been shown by prospective studies in patients with acute myocardial infarction, cerebrovascular accident and in immobilized general medical patients.

ACUTE MYOCARDIAL INFARCTION (AMI). Patients not receiving anticoagulant therapy as a primary treatment of AMI are at risk for venous thromboembolism. The recommended prophylaxis is low dose heparin or LMWH.

STROKE. Patients with ischaemic stroke are at high risk for venous thromboembolism. The recommended prophylaxis is low dose heparin, LMWH or low molecular weight heparinoid.

IMMOBILIZED GENERAL MEDICAL PATIENTS. Patients at risk should receive prophylaxis. The following modalities could be considered:

- Graduated compression stockings;
- Intermittent pneumatic compression;
- Low dose heparin;
- LMWH;
- Low molecular weight heparinoid;
- Oral anticoagulants.

PATIENTS AT RISK FOR THROMBOEMBOLISM; DEFINING RISK CATEGORIES AND APPLICATION OF COMBINED METHODS OF PROPHYLAXIS. It is possible to categorize patients in risk groups using clinical criteria, which have been shown to be associated with a risk of venous thromboembolism (Tables 11.3–11.5).

COMBINED FORMS OF PROPHYLAXIS

Surgery

High risk patients. All high risk patients should receive prophylaxis. Apart from single modalities that have been demonstrated to be effective and safe, such as low dose heparin and LMWH, combined modalities may be considered for local practice, i.e. combinations of pharmacological and mechanical methods such as low dose heparin or LMWH combined with mechanical methods.

Table 11.3. Risk categories in surgical patients.

Risk category	Risk of venous thromboembolism (assessed by objective tests)		
	Calf vein DVT	Proximal DVT	Fatal PE
High risk			
General/urological surgery in patients over 40 years with recent history of DVT or PE	40–80	10–30	1–5
Extensive pelvic or abdominal surgery for malignant disease			
Major orthopaedic surgery of lower limbs			
Moderate risk			
General surgery in patients >40 years lasting 30 min or more and in patients <40 years on oral contraceptives	10–40	2–10	0.1–0.7
Low risk			
Uncomplicated surgery in patients <40 years without additional risk factors	<10	<1	<0.01
Minor surgery (<30 min) in patients >40 years without additional risk factors			

Table 11.4. Risk categories in gynaecology and obstetrics.

	Gynaecology	Obstetrics
High risk	History of previous DVT/PE	History of previous DVT/PE
	Age >60	
	Cancer	
	Thrombophilic condition	Thrombophilic condition
Moderate risk	Patients over 40 years with major surgery	Advanced age of over 40 years
	Patients below 40 years on oral contraceptives with major surgery	
Low risk	Uncomplicated surgery <40 years without additional risk factors	*
	Minor surgery (<30 min)	
	Patients over 40 years without additional risk factors	

*The risk of DVT in obstetric patients with pre-eclampsia and other risk factors is unknown but prophylaxis should be considered.

Table 11.5. Risk categories in medical patients.

High risk	• Stroke
	• Congestive heart failure
	• Thrombophilia with additional disease
Moderate/low risk	• All immobilized patients with active disease (risk increased by infectious diseases, malignancy and other risk factors)

Moderate risk patients. Combined mechanical methods may be applied as an alternative to low dose heparin or LMWH.

Gynaecology patients. Combinations of prophylaxis have not been evaluated properly in patients but, on the basis of results of other surgical trials, combined prophylaxis may be considered.

Medical patients. In particular, in high risk patients there is a lack of studies employing combined methods in the prevention of DVT/PE. Hence, no specific recommendations regarding the application of combined prevention modalities can be provided.

COST-EFFECTIVENESS FOR ALL GROUPS. In discussing the prophylactic methods used in the prevention of thromboembolism, it is important to consider health economics. Primary prevention is more cost-effective than secondary prevention through routine screening of postoperative patients.

In *medium and high risk patients*, the costs following thromboembolism are so high that the currently recommended methods of primary prophylaxis are very cost-effective.

In *low risk patients*, no data are available at present concerning the cost-effectiveness of the current recommended prophylactic methods.

SECONDARY PREVENTION. The objectives of treatment of thromboembolism are to prevent extension of the thrombus, progressive swelling of the leg resulting in increased compartmental pressure which can lead to phlegmasia caerulea dolens, venous gangrene and limb loss. Also, the recurrence of thrombosis and/or PE, which can be fatal or later lead to chronic pulmonary hypertension, must be prevented. Finally, the prevention should avoid the progression to the post-thrombotic syndrome by preservation of the venous outflow and functional valves.

ANTICOAGULANTS are necessary for reducing morbidity and mortality due to DVT/PE. Anticoagulation should be started either with an initial course of intravenous adjusted dose standard heparin given by continuous infusion or with subcutaneous adjusted dose standard heparin. It is important that therapeutic level is reached within the first 24 hours. APTT should be at least 1.5 times the patient's control value, which usually requires an initial i.v. bolus injection. APTT measurements in patients treated with subcutaneous heparin should be done in the mid-interval after two injections. The upper limit for

APTT varies according to local practice and is not well defined. The heparin regimen should be continued for a minimum period of 5–7 days.

It is acceptable to start oral anticoagulant therapy on the first day of heparin therapy or on subsequent days. Under normal circumstances, heparin treatment should be interrupted when the patient's INR is within the therapeutic range (i.e. 2–3) for at least two days. Oral anticoagulant therapy should be continued for a period of at least three months in patients with a first episode of DVT and no continuing risk factors. However, the optimal duration of therapy is not known. Patients presenting with a recurrent episode of DVT should be treated with heparin with the same therapeutic regimen as for patients with a first episode of DVT. However, the duration of oral anticoagulant therapy is not known. Adjusted doses of subcutaneous heparin may be used as secondary prophylaxis in special clinical conditions such as pregnancy and other contraindications to oral anticoagulant therapy.

LMWHs given subcutaneously have been shown to be as effective as standard heparin for the initial treatment of DVT in terms of reduction of the thrombus size as assessed by repeated venograpy. Preliminary results demonstrate that LMWHs are as effective as adjusted dose intravenous standard heparin in the prevention of symptomatic recurrent venous thromboembolism during long term follow-up. There is good evidence that thrombolytic therapy produces a more effective lysis in proximal DVT than unfractionated heparin, but its use is limited because the benefit–risk ratio of this treatment as compared with unfractionated heparin has not yet been established.

Thus, there is currently insufficient evidence that all patients with DVT require thrombolytic therapy. Thrombolytic treatment may be considered in selected patients who suffer from recent massive DVT in the absence of contraindications.

Thrombectomy is indicated for limb salvage (phlegmasia, impending venous gangrene) but its use under other circumstances is limited.

A filter device should be inserted in the inferior vena cava when anticoagulation is contraindicated in the management of PE or DVT above the knee or when adequate anticoagulation fails to prevent recurrent thromboembolism. For thrombosis extending to or involving the renal veins and in pregnant patients, a prospectively proved device (i.e. Greenfield filter) should be placed above the level of the renal veins.

UNRESOLVED ISSUES

- The risk for DVT/PE continues beyond hospitalization. It needs to be assessed in prospective trials considering the need to continue prophylaxis beyond hospitalization.
- There is a need for a proper randomized comparison of pre- and postoperative commencement of pharmacological prophylactic modalities.
- In moderate risk patients it is important to compare fixed low dose heparin with LMWH (mortality and confirmed fatal PE).
- Further studies are needed to see whether graduated stockings and/or IPC enhance the efficacy of pharmacological methods.
- A prospective register (postmarketing surveillance) on the prevalence of spinal (epidural) anaesthesia-induced haemorrhage in patients pretreated with DVT/PE prophylactic anticoagulants is needed.
- It is important to establish the risk of DVT in large series of laparoscopic abdominal surgical procedures.
- There is a need for multicentre trials comparing standard heparin with LMWH in high risk pregnant patients, assessing safety, efficacy and side effects such as oteoporosis.

CHAPTER 12

VARICOCOELE

Diagnosis

- Enlarged veins in the spermatic cord (usually left)
- Pain, tension at the left hemiscrotum
- Reflux in the spermatic veins
- Infertility in some patients

Introduction

Varicocoele means varicosities of the pampiniform plexus. It is due to incompetence or absence of valves in the spermatic and testicular vein (Figure 12.1). The hydrostatic venous pressure is transmitted to the spermatic cord causing distension and tortuosity of the pampiniform plexus. Most often (90%) varicocoele is present on the left side where the termination of the spermatic vein into the left renal vein allows more direct transmission of retrograde pressure along the incompetent vein to the scrotum. In the case of a gross varicocoele the spermatic cord is distended by multiple veins which are visible and palpable. The definition of varicocoele implies that there is venous incompetence allowing reflux of blood from the great veins into the plexus.

It is possible to have dilated veins without incompetence and vice versa. Clinically overt varicocoele is easy to diagnose and evaluate and enlarged veins may be palpated with the patient standing and are often said to feel like a "bag of worms". If the patient is only examined lying down then the diagnosis may be missed. The testis appears enlarged and patients may complain of a dragging scrotal sensation. Mild, asymptomatic varicocoele

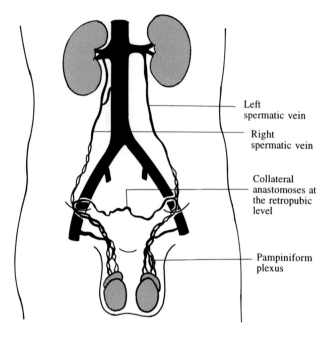

Figure 12.1

may be unassociated with signs/symptoms and difficult to detect clinically. Varicocoele in its clinical and subclinical forms is considered to be a possible, important cause of male infertility, especially if bilateral. Sudden onset of varicocoele in the older patient may be caused by an obstruction of the left renal vein by a carcinoma of the kidney. If suspected an ultrasound scan will usually confirm the diagnosis.

The diagnosis of varicocoele is now usually made with ultrasound. B-mode ultrasound scanning indicates the presence of dilated veins, increasing in size during a Valsalva manoeuvre or by standing. Colour duplex scanning visualizes the veins and demonstrates retrograde reflux. Reflux in the spermatic plexus is first evaluated and shown with the patient supine, fully relaxed, performing a Valsalva manoeuvre (Figure 12.2). The reflux in the spermatic plexus is visible during Valsalva. Reflux is often transmitted distally to the veins surrounding the testis. In case there is no demonstrable reflux in the supine position, the test may be repeated whith the patient standing.

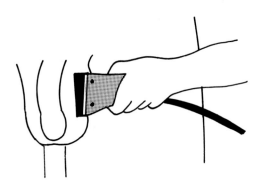

Figure 12.2

Phlebography is still widely used to demonstrate varicocoele. Often, during the diagnostic procedure a sclerosing agent may be injected.

Symptomatic varicocoele is usually treated surgically with ligation of the spermatic vein at or above the internal inguinal ring. All testicular veins but one are ligated. The procedure may also be performed with laparoscopy.

Asymptomatic varicocoele usually requires no treatment.

Recurrent varicocoele and asymptomatic varicocoele associated with significant reflux (> 3 sec) on colour duplex may be treated with transfemoral catheterization of the left spermatic vein by retrograde injection of sclerosing agents into the vein. Also, occlusion of the spermatic vein may be obtained with a detachable ballon inserted by femoral vein catheterization.

The long term results of treatments are usually very satisfactory. It has been observed that an increase in sperm count may be observed in subjects with low fertility after treatment of the varicocoele and therefore the screening and treatment of varicocoele should always be considered in infertility.

CHAPTER 13

THE PELVIC CONGESTION SYNDROME AND VULVAR VARICES

Diagnosis

- Pelvic pain
- Vulvar varicosities
- Ovarian vein reflux

Introduction

The pelvic congestion syndrome (PCS) is often unrecognized or poorly treated, and patients are treated by different specialists for the two main problems present: pelvic pain and vulvar varicosities. Vulvar varicose veins are a relatively common disorder, sometimes associated with pelvic pain, but they are not necessarily related to PCS. The anatomy of the ovarian veins is shown in Figure 13.1. Vulvar varicosity may be associated [Figure 13.1(b)] with:

* True varicocoele (reflux in the ovarian vein, particularly the left one (A);
* Secondary venous distension due to iliac or pelvic obstruction (B);
* Severe reflux and venous hypertension at the level of the femoral vein, long saphenous vein and its medial collaterals;
* Localized varicosities associated with cavernosal tissue and sometimes with small arterio-venous communications.

The aetiology of vulvar varicose veins has been considered to be an equivalent to post-thrombotic syndrome in the legs. Following pregnancy some of the divisions of the internal iliac veins may occlude and the resulting

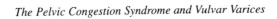

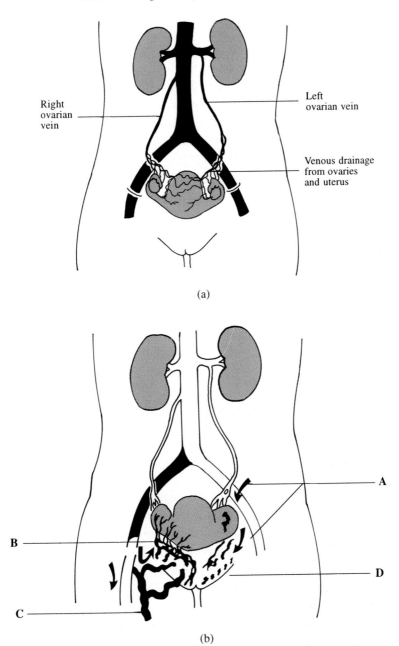

(a)

(b)

Figure 13.1

outflow obstruction produces signs and symptoms similar to the post-thrombotic syndrome in the leg. Perivulvar varices are common during pregnancy, but they usually disappear after delivery. The sudden appearance of vulvar varicose veins during the third or fourth month of the second or third pregnancy may indicate a pelvic vein thrombosis. In some patients vulvar varices persist and increase in size with subsequent pregnancies. They may extend to the posterior part of the leg and thigh. It is possible that PCS is associated with consequences of a DVT, but it is also possible that simple, pure ovarian vein reflux may be the basis of the disorder.

PCS is characterized by *pain* of variable intensity which is worse premenstrually, and it is increased by fatigue, standing, and during or after intercourse. These symptoms are often associated with vulvar varicosities. Also, "broad ligament varicocoele" (Lefevre, 1964) has been associated with chronic pelvic pain in multiparous women. Pelvic varicosities exist when the ovarian veins are congenitally incompetent, causing a situation which is analogous to scrotal varicocoele in men.

Diagnosis

On examination of patients with PCS, atypical veins are seen to be present on the back of the thigh arising from the posterior vulvar area. The vulvar varicosities may be in communication with the long saphenous vein, which may be filled from the posterior vulvar veins.

True ovarian varicocoele may be diagnosed with ultrasound, or phlebography. A congested ovary may be shown by ultrasound, and reflux in the ovarian veins may be observed by colour Duplex — but only in some patients — during Valsalva. The dilated ovarian vein may be demonstrated by direct vulvar venography (Hobbs) or by retrograde phlebography. It is important to exclude other inflammatory conditions (including Crohn's disease, diverticulosis and tumours), vertebral problems causing neural compression as well as genito-urinary diseases (ovarian cysts, endometriosis, tumours, etc.).

Localized vulvar veins (particularly in young subjects) may be a separate clinical entity. Cavernosal tissue may also be present (Figure 13.2). Colour and power duplex show the diffuse reticular vascular structure not related to ovarian reflux.

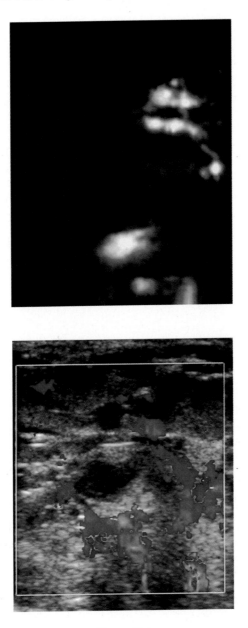

Figure 13.2

The treatment of PCS may be conservative (suppression of ovarian function) or surgical (retroperitoneal ligation of the veins, ovariectomy or even hysterectomy). Sclerotherapy of the vulvar veins has also been used using 3% STD, with good results. Retrograde catheterization and sclerosis of the ovarian vein have also been attempted. If untreated, PCS often tends to disappear after the menopause.

CHAPTER 14

HAEMORRHOIDS

Diagnosis

- Rectal bleeding, protrusion, discomfort, mucoid discharge from rectum, pruritus ani
- Secondary anaemia
- Characteristic findings on external anal inspection and anoscopic examination

Introduction

Haemorrhoids (piles) are a normal anatomic state, and only when they become enlarged and signs and symptoms are present is treatment indicated.

Internal haemorroids (plexus of the superior hemorrhoidal veins above the muscolocutaneous junction) are covered by mucosa. Haemorrhoids may occur in three primary positions: right anterior, right posterior and left lateral (Figure 14.1). Smaller haemorrhoids may occur between these primary locations.

External haemorrhoids (inferior haemorrhoidal plexus) occur below the mucocutaneous junction in the tissue beneath the anal epithelium of the anal canal and the skin of the perianal region. The two plexuses of internal and external haemorrhoids anastomose freely and include the venous return from the lower rectum and anus. Internal haemorrhoids drain to the superior haemorrhoidal veins and to the portal vein system. External haemorroids drain into the systemic circulation. Haemorrhoids become symptomatic for different reasons, including straining in the squatting position, which increases venous pressure, distending the veins and facilitating protrusion and bleeding. Other factors considered to be important are chronic constipation, pregnancy,

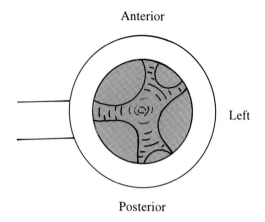

Figure 14.1

obesity and a low fibre diet (imposing increased venous pressure during defecation). They are much more common in the western world than in undeveloped countries.

Diagnosis

Most haemorrhoids are asymptomatic. Severe pain is associated only with thrombosis of external haemorrhoids and does not usually occur with internal haemorrhoids. Bleeding is usually the first indication of internal haemorrhoids. The blood is bright red, not mixed with stools, and is variable in quantity. Recurrent bleeding may lead to anaemia. Only rarely is bleeding profuse and life-threatening. As haemorrhoids enlarge they may prolapse, at first only with defecation followed by spontaneous reduction, while later the patient may be forced to manually replace the haemorrhoids. At the final stage they may be permanently prolapsed. Pain and discomfort are usually associated with complications such as thrombosis, oedema and inflammation. Pruritus ani is also a common complaint.

On examination external haemorrhoids are seen with inspection, particularly when thrombosed. Internal haemorrhoids may prolapse when the patient is asked to strain. On digital rectal examination internal haemorrhoids cannot usually be palpated and they should not be tender. Anoscopic examination demonstrates internal haemorrhoids which do not prolapse. Gentle straining from the patient shows the size and degree of the prolapse. Proctosigmoidoscopy is needed to exclude inflammatory or neoplastic disease at higher level.

Classification

First degree, internal haemorrhoids are usually painless but may be associated with bleeding during defecation. Usually at this stage there is no prolapse and anoscopy shows enlarged haemorrhoids projecting into the lumen.

Second degree haemorrhoids protrude through the anal canal on gentle straining. They usually reduce spontaneously after straining or defecation.

Third degree haemorrhoids protrude with straining and must be reduced manually after defecation.

Fourth degree haemorrhoids are associated with permanent protrusion and usually with local complications such as oedema, inflammation and mucous discharge.

Differential Diagnosis

The most common sign of haemorrhoids, rectal bleeding, occurs also with neoplastic diseases, adenomatous polyps, diverticular disease and inflammatory disorders. Barium enema and colonscopy should be performed when needed, particularly in older patients, to exclude more severe problems. Procidentia (rectal prolapse) is differentiated from mucosal prolapse due to internal haemorrhoids, as in the former condition a circle of protruding bowel appears. This involves the full thickness of the bowel wall with concentric mucosal folds. The double full thickness of the wall is perceived by digital palpation. Haemorrhoids and rectal prolapse may coexist. Other perianal lesions and anorectal tumours are characteristic in their appearance. Thrombosed external haemorrhoids are described in the following section. External skin tags may indicate previous thrombosis of external haemorrhoids while the presence of a midline sentinel tag may indicate the presence of an anal fissure.

Complications

Occasionally, prolapsed haemorrhoids become irreducible as the consequence of congestion, oedema and/or thrombosis. This is usually associated with severe pain and may result in infarction of the overlying mucosa and skin. Anaemia is a relatively common condition complicating haemorrhoids. A rare complication is septic embolization into the portal system, which may cause liver abscesses. In patients with portal hypertension, bleeding may be very profuse as haemorrhoids may act as a portal venous to systemic venous shunt.

Treatment

The main aim of treatment is to control symptoms. Treatment is therefore based on the clinical presentation.

Conservative medical treatment is used in first and second degree haemorrhoids (diet high in fibres, increased water intake, hydrophylic agents to increase dietary bulk). Prolapsed thrombosed haemorrhoids are treated with gentle reduction, rest and local treatment to decrease local inflammation and swelling. Emergency surgery is not usually performed because of the risk of portal pyaemia.

Injection treatment (sclerotherapy) is used for first and second degree haemorrhoids. A haemorrhoidal needle is used to inject through an anoscope above the mucocutaneous junction. The sclerosing agent (i.e. 5% phenol in vegetable oil) is injected submucosally into the loose areolar tissue above the internal haemorrhoids. Inflammation and scarring occur after injection, resulting in shrinkage of the haemorrhoid. If placed above the dentate line the injections are usually painless and can be repeated on an out-patient basis.

Rubber band ligation can be used for prolapsed and enlarged haemorrhoids. With an anoscope the redundant mucosa above the haemorrhoidal plexus is grasped and advanced through a special ligator. The rubber band causes ischaemic necrosis followed by fibrosis and fixation of the tissues. After treatment in some patients pain may be severe and require the removal of the band.

By *cryosurgery* haemorrhoids are necrosed by freezing the tissue with a cryoprobe (CO_2 or N_2O). The method is not very diffuse, and delayed wound healing may occur.

Surgery (haemorroidectomy) is used for patients with severe, chronic symptoms and third or fourth degree prolapse. These subjects are often anaemic and do not respond well to conservative treatments. Correct surgery consists in excision of the redundant tissue with conservative excision of normal anoderm and skin particularly avoiding damage to the underlying sphincter. Surgical treatment may also be performed using a surgical laser.

Other treatments include anal dilatation (to disrupt bands of the anal canal), infrared photocoagulation, bipolar diathermy and other out-patient-based methods. Their rate of success is not clear.

Thrombosed External Haemorrhoids

Thrombosed external haemorrhoids are characterized by a painful, tense, bluish mass or elevation beneath the skin or anoderm caused by a thrombosis of the subcutaneous external haemorrhoidal veins of the anal canal. It is more appropriately considered a perianal haematoma. Thrombosis of an external haemorrhoid usually follows a sudden increase in abdominal pressure (heavy lifting, coughing, sneezing, straining during defecation). It generally affects young healthy subjects and it is not directly related to internal haemorrhoids. Immediate relief may be obtained by evacuation of the thrombus or complete excision (external haemorrhoidectomy) if the patient is examined within the first 48 hours. An elipse of skin should also be removed to prevent re-formation of the underlying clot. When the thrombus is organized conservative measures are more appropriate.

CHAPTER 15

ABNORMAL ARTERIOVENOUS COMMUNICATIONS (FISTULAS)

Diagnosis

- Continuous "machinery" murmur, palpable thrill and (rarely) decrease in heart rate with compression of the fistula (Branham's sign)
- Increased heart rate, signs/symptoms of increased cardiac output, heart failure
- Dilated and/or varicose veins

Introduction and General Considerations

Abnormal arteriovenous (AV) communications (fistulas) may be congenital or acquired and may affect vessels of all sizes. Their effects depend upon the quantity of blood shunting. In *congenital fistulas*, the systemic effect is often not great, because the degree of communication, though diffuse, is usually small. Larger, *acquired fistulas* enlarge rapidly. Cardiac dilatation and failure result when shunting is excessive, prolonged and/or untreated. AV fistulas have also been considered as one of the abnormalities present and determining the occurrence of varicose veins (Shalin). Small congenital fistulas are often noted in infancy or childhood. When a limb is involved, muscle mass or bone length may be increased. AV malformations may involve the brain, visceral organs, or lungs. Gastrointestinal haemorrhage may occur while pulmonary lesions cause polycythaemia, clubbing and cyanosis.

Acquired fistulas usually result from injuries that produce artificial connections between adjacent arteries and veins and may be the result of trauma or disease. Penetrating injuries are the most common cause, but fistulas are sometimes seen after blunt trauma.

Iatrogenic AV fistulas after arteriography are becoming increasingly common. *Connective tissue disorders* (e.g. Ehlers–Danlos syndrome), erosion of an atherosclerotic or mycotic arterial *aneurysm* into adjacent veins, communication with an arterial prosthetic graft, and *neoplastic invasion* are other causes.

A rare but dramatic cause of atraumatic AV fistula is *combined injury to the aorta and inferior vena cava or to the iliac arteries and veins during surgical excision of a herniated nucleus pulposus* by the dorsal approach.

Clinical Findings

Signs and symptoms

The time of onset and the presence or absence of associated disease should be determined. A typical continuous "machinery" murmur can be heard over most fistulas and is often associated with a palpable thrill and locally increased skin temperature. Proximally, the arteries and veins dilate and the pulse distal to the lesion diminishes. The limb, distally to the communication, may be cooler. There may be varicose veins or signs of venous insufficiency. Tachycardia occurs in some subjects as a consequence of increased cardiac output and right ventricle overload.

When the fistula is occluded by manual compression or by compression with an ultrasound probe, the pulse rate tends to slow (Branham's sign).

Imaging studies

Noninvasive investigations (colour duplex scanning) are very effective in imaging the fistulas and their connections. Occasionally it is possible to quantify the blood flow. Typical low resistance waveforms (with high diastolic component) and high velocity are demonstrated in most patients. In the most severe cases the venous flow is completely modified from a waveform phasic with respiration to a continuous high velocity pattern.

Magnetic resonance imaging (MRI) has an important role in the evaluation and follow-up of arteriovenous malformations. The precise demonstration of larger AV fistulas is completed with selective arteriography. This procedure is indicated when surgery or embolization is planned.

Treatment

Only some AV connections require treatment. Small peripheral fistulas may constitute a cosmetic problem, but if there is no severe associated sign a conservative approach is indicated. Also, many fistulas are too diffuse, too small or too deep to be surgically accessible.

Indications for surgery or radiological intervention include haemorrhagic complications, expanding false aneurysm, severe venous or arterial insufficiency, important cosmetic deformity and, only in a limited number of patients, heart failure. Many fistulas are now managed by the interventional radiologist with embolization under angiography control. The fistulas are embolized from the arterial sector. Several types of embolic material have been used (i.e. gelfoam, blood clots, glass beads and part of muscle tissue). Good results have been documented with AV malformations in different anatomical districts. Intracranial arteriovenous malformations and all fistulas of the head and neck appear better suited for this form of therapy, which has the advantage of being repeatable.

Surgical treatment theoretically includes ligation of all major feeding arteries and draining veins. However, the procedure is most often incomplete and recurrence after some time is frequent, particularly in congenital malformations. Amputation of the extermity, *en bloc* resection of the tissue including the fistula, and repair of the fistula by reconstruction of the involved arteries and veins, are also used. Oversewing the defects in the artery and vein is curative for postarteriography fistulas.

Congenital AV fistulas are amenable to surgical management only when *en bloc* resection of all tissue involved in the fistula can be accomplished. When the AV connections involve several portions of an extremity, local arterial ligation is invariably followed by recurrence, and only temporary palliation can be expected. Often the involved venous structures in a limb do not resemble actual veins but a sort of venous lakes limited by endothelium which are very difficult to isolate and ligate.

Rarely, amputation may be a last resort to control unmanageable peripheral fistulas.

Sclerotherapy may be used in the treatment of minor venous dilatations (after arterial ligation).

Prognosis

The results of therapy vary according to the extent, location and type of fistula. In general, traumatic fistulas have a favourable prognosis and technically they are often corrected without problems. Congenital fistulas are very difficult to treat, as several connections are usually found and only some are visible in the operating field. There is a high possibility of recurrence with these fistulas and indications for surgery are usually limited to the most urgent cases.

Primary Aortocaval Fistulas

Spontaneous aortocaval fistulas between an abdominal aortic aneurysm and the inferior vena cava are a complication seen in some 1–2% of patients treated for abdominal aortic aneurysm and 5–6% of patients with a ruptured aortic aneurysm. The fistula is often misdiagnosed before surgery for ruptured aortic aneurysm but specific signs (i.e. a pulsating abdominal mass, continuous "machinery" murmur, high output, hyperdynamic heart failure) may be present.

Often fistulas between the vena cava and the aneurysm are symptom-free or the signs are not evident in an already complex clinical picture and are a surgical surprise. Pulmonary embolism in these patients is rare.

Surgery is the treatment of choice for most patients with aortocaval fistulas, usually in combination with aortic aneurysm repair.

Surgical repair after careful dissection of the iliac veins and the cava is possible. Digital control of the AV communication and endoaneuryismal repair of the fistula have been accomplished with a high mortality rate (35–40%), mainly due to multiple organ failure.

The *prognosis* is generally poor, particularly if the communication is not detected and surgery is delayed or not possible.

CHAPTER 16

DRUGS AND TREATMENTS USED IN VENOUS DISEASES

The drugs used in venous diseases may be divided into four main groups:

(1) Drugs used for DVT prophylaxis
(2) Drugs used for DVT treatment
(3) Drugs used for venous insufficiency
(4) Drugs used for sclerotherapy

These drugs may be classified according to their mechanisms of action (Table 16.1).

The most important *physical methods* used to treat venous diseases are:

(1) Elastic compression stockings
(2) Bandages
(3) Pneumatic (simple or sequential compression)

Anticoagulants

The main use of anticoagulants is to prevent thrombus formation or extension of an existing thrombus. Prevention is mainly directed to stopping the progression of venous thrombi consisting of a fibrin web enmeshed with platelets and red cells. Anticoagulants are widely used in the prevention and treatment of DVT, particularly in the leg.

Heparin is defined as *standard* or *unfractionated*, in contrast with *low dose* and *low molecular weight heparins (LMWH)*. Heparin initiates anticoagulation rapidly but has a short duration of action. For the initial treatment of DVT and PE an intravenous loading dose is followed by continuous intravenous infusion (using an infusion pump) or by intermittent

Table 16.1. Drugs used in venous diseases.

(1) *Anticoagulants and protamine*
    Parenteral anticoagulants
        Heparin
        Low molecular weight heparin (LMWH)
        Ancrod
        Epoprostenol
    Protamine
(2) *Oral anticoagulants*
        Warfarin
        Nicoumalone
        Phenidione
(3) *Antiplatelet drugs*
        Aspirin
        Dipyridamole
        Ticlopidine
        Indobufen
        Others
(4) *Fibrinolytic drugs*
        Alteplase (rt-PA, tissue type plasminogen activator)
        Streptokinase
        Urokinase
(5) *Other drugs used for DVT and PE prophylaxis*
        Dextran
        Heparinoids/antithrombotics
(6) *"Venoactive" drugs*
        Daflon 500
        Centellase
        Venoruton-Paroven
        Troxerutin
        Meliven
        Others
(7) *Drugs used for venous ulcerations*
        Defibrotide
        Pentoxiphyllin
(8) *Heparinoids*
        Mesoglycan
        Orgaran
        Defibrotide

subcutaneous injection. The use of intermittent intravenous injection is no longer recommended. An oral anticoagulant (usually warfarin) is started at the same time or a few hours after heparin (which needs to be continued for at least three days or until the the oral anticoagulant has taken effect). Daily laboratory monitoring is essential. Determination of APTT (activated partial thromboplastin time) is the most widely used method.

Low dose heparin by subcutaneous injection is widely used for prevention of DVT and PE in high risk patients. Laboratory monitoring is not required with this standard prophylactic regimen.

An *adjusted dose regimen (with monitoring)* or *LMWH* is used in major orthopaedic surgery (which has a high risk of DVT and PE).

Complications. Haemorrage is the most common complication. Heparin treatment is usually discontinued. When a rapid reversal of heparin anticoagulation is needed, protamine sulphate is the specific antidote.

Cautions. The platelet count must be checked in patients treated for more than five days. Heparin should be stopped immediately in patients developing thrombocytopenia.

Contraindications are haemophilia, haemorragic disorders, thrombocytopenia, active peptic ulcer, cerebral aneurysm, severe liver disease, recent surgery of the eye or nervous system, severe hypertension, and hypersensitivity to heparin.

Side effects are haemorrage, skin necrosis, thrombocitopenia, hypersensitivity reactions, osteoporosis (after prolonged use), alopecia.

Treatment of DVT and PE. A loading intravenous injection (5000 units or 10 000 in severe PE) of heparin is administered followed by continuous infusion (1000–2000 units/hr or by subcutaneous injection of 15 000 units every 12 hours (both adjusted daily by laboratory monitoring). In small adults/children a lower loading dose is used, then 15–25 units/kg/hr intravenously or 250 units/kg every 12 hours by subcutaneous injections.

Prophylaxis of DVT and PE. Subcutaneous injections are given (5000 units, 2 hours before surgery, then every 8–12 hours for 7 days or until the patient is ambulant). With this method monitoring is not needed. During pregnancy (with monitoring) 10 000 units are given every 12 hours. For the prevention of thrombosis of prostetic heart valves, subcutaneous heparin is given every

12 hours and adjusted to prolong the APTT to 1–1.5 times the control value 6 hours after the last injection.

LMWHs are as effective and safe as unfractionated heparin in the prevention of DVT and PE. In orthopaedic surgery they are probably more effective. Their duration of action is longer than unfractionated heparin. They are generally used once daily and the standard prophylactic regimen does not require monitoring. The effects of LMWHs are only partially reversed by protamine. Different dosages are used with different LMWHs, as the fractions in the compounds differ in quantity and quality. Also, different compounds are available in different countries. Specific instructions must be observed and the prophylaxis dosage cannot be generalized.

Protamine sulphate is used to counteract the action of heparin. *Side effects* include flushing, hypotension and bradycardia.

Dose (by slow intravenous injection): 1 mg neutralizes 100 units of heparin (mucous) or 80 units of heparin (lung) when given within 15 minutes. If heparin has been given a long time before protamine, less protamine is required as heparin is rapidly excreted. The maximum dose is 50 mg.

Ancrod reduces plasma fibrinogen by cleavage of fibrin.

Indications are DVT, prevention of postoperative thrombosis ("named patient" basis only).

Cautions, contraindications and side effects are similar to those described for heparin. Resistance may develop. Administration with dextran must be avoided.

Dose: intravenous infusion: 2–3 units/kg over 4–12 hours (usually 6–8 hours), then by infusion or slow intravenous injection 2 units/kg every 12 hours. By subcutaneous injection Ancrod is used for prophylaxis of DVT at the dose of 280 units immediately after surgery, then 70 units daily for 4 days (i.e. fractured femur) or 8 days (i.e. hip replacement).

Note: the initial infusion must be slow to avoid massive intravascular formation of unstable fibrin. Response is monitored observing clot size after the blood has been allowed to stand for two hours. Plasma fibrinogen concentration can also be directly measured.

Complications: the most frequent are haemorrhages. As it takes 12–24 hours for haemostatic fibrinogen concentrations to be restored after stopping administration, it may be necessary to give Ancrod antivenom (Arvin Antidote;

0.2 mL test dose subcutaneously followed by 0.8 mL intramuscularly and 30 minutes later 1 mL intravenously). The antivenom may cause anaphylaxis. As an alternative, reconstituted freeze-dried fibrinogen or fresh frozen plasma may be given.

Epoprostenol is mainly used to inhibit platelet aggregation during renal dialysis, either alone or with heparin. Its half-life is very short (3 minutes), and therefore it must be given by continuous intravenous infusion. It is a potent vasodilatator and therefore side effects include flushing, headache and hypotension. Anticoagulant monitoring is required when it is administered with heparin.

Oral anticoagulants (OAs) antagonize the effects of vitamin K. OAs take about 48–72 hours to develop their full anticoagulant effect. When immediate anticoagulation is needed heparin is given simultaneously. The main indication for OAs is DVT and PE. OAs should not be used in patients with recent cerebral thrombosis.

Warfarin is generally considered the drug of choice. Nicoumalone and phenidione are seldom used. The baseline prothrombin time (PT) should be determined before the initial dose is given. The usual adult induction dose of warfarin is 10 mg daily for 2 days. The subsequent maintenance dose is considered on the basis of PT (reported as INR). The recommended therapeutic ranges are:

- INR 2–2.5 for DVT prophylaxis including surgery on high risk patients.
- INR 2–3 for hip surgery, fractured femur operations, treatment of DVT or PE.
- INR 3–4.5 for recurrent DVT or PE.

INR is determined daily or on alternate days in the early days of treatment, then at longer intervals (depending on response), and then up to 6–8 weeks. The daily maintenance dose of warfarin is 3–9 mg (taken at the same time each day). The most common *complication* of OAs is haemorrage. The dose is omitted and the INR checked. On the basis of the INR treatment is established (vitamin K1, concentrate of factor II.IX,X and VII in the most severe cases). When the INR is 4.5–7 the treatment is discontinued, and when the INR is >7 without haemorrage warfarin is discontinued and vitamin K_1 is given. When unexpected bleeding occurs at therapeutic levels, unrecognized or subclinical disease (i.e. ulcerative bowel disease) is usually present.

A devastating complication of oral anticoagulant therapy is haemorrhagic skin necrosis, which in the past was considered to be an allergic reaction. However, patients with this complication are deficient in protein C, which may be the predisposing factor.

OAs in pregnancy. OAs may damage the foetus and should not be given in the first trimester of pregnancy. Women at risk of pregnancy should stop warfarin. OAs also cross the placenta, causing risk of placental and foetal haemorrhage. Therefore they should be avoided during pregnancy. Difficult decisions have to be made in women with prosthetic heart valves who have a history of recent DVT or PE.

Warfarin is indicated mainly for secondary prophylaxis and treatment of DVT and PE.

Cautions: hepatic and renal disease, recent surgery interactions with other drugs.

Contraindications: pregnancy, ulcerative disease, severe hypertension, bacterial endocarditis.

Side effects: haemorrhage.

Dose: as indicated above.

Nicoumalone (Sinthrome).The same indications, cautions, contraindications and side effects of warfarin should be observed. This drug should be avoided during breast-feeding.

Dose: 8–10 mg on the first day; 4–8 mg on the second day; maintenance dose usually 1–8 mg daily.

Phenidione (Dindevan). The same indications, cautions, contraindications and side effects of warfarin should be observed. Side effects include hypersensitivity reactions. This drug should also be avoided during breast-feeding.

Dose: 200 mg on the first day; 100 mg on the second day; maintenance dose usually 50–150 mg daily.

Antiplatelet Drugs

Antiplatelet drugs inhibit thrombus formation on the arterial side of the circulation where thrombi are formed by platelet aggregation and anticoagulants have little effect. Antiplatelet drugs have little effect in venous thromboebolism. So far only *aspirin* has been used extensively in practice but no significant results have been obtained by aspirin prophylaxis of DVT and PE. Therefore the role of aspirin in the prophylaxis of venous thromboembolism remains uncertain.

Indobufen prophylaxis (200 mg bid, after 6-month anticoagulation) has reduced in a prospective, three-year study the incidence of recurrent DVT after a major thrombotic episode of the lower limbs. However, the experience with this drug is limited.

Fibrinolytic Drugs

These drugs activate plasminogen to form plasmin which degrades fibrin, promoting the lysis of thrombi.

Caution. There is a risk of bleeding from venepuncture or surgical wounds, and a risk of embolization from the clot.

Contraindications are recent haemorrhage, trauma, surgery, dental procedures, coagulation defects, cerebrovascular disease, intestinal ulcerations, gynaecological problems causing bleeding, pulmonary disease with cavitation, acute pancreatitis, diabetic rethinopathy, severe liver disease and oesophageal varices.

Side effects of thrombolytic drugs are nausea, vomiting and back pain. Bleeding is usually limited at the site of injection but serious haemorrage (i.e. cerebral) has been reported. With serious bleeding treatment should be discontinued and administration of coagulation factors or antifibrinolytic drugs (aprotinin, tranexamic acid) may be required. Streptokinase and anistreplase may cause allergic reactions and anaphylaxis.

Alteplase (rt-PA, tissue plasminogen activator) and *Anistreplase* are indicated mainly for acute myocardial infarction, and are used for PE (10 mg by intravenous injection in 2 minutes + 90 mg in 2 hours).

Streptokinase (Kabikinase, Streptase) is used for myocardial infarction and is also indicated for DVT and PE.

Dose: by intravenous infusion 250 000 units over 30 minutes, then 100 000 units every hour for up to 24–72 hours according to the clinical problem (see data sheet).

Urokinase (Ukidan, Urokinase) is used for thrombosed AV and intravenous cannulas, thrombolysis in the eye, DVT and PE.

Dose: by intravenous infusion 4400 international units/kg over 10 minutes, then 4400 units/kg/hour for 12 hours in PE or 12–24 hours in DVT. For bolus injection in PE see data sheet.

Other drugs used in the prophylaxis of DVT and PE are Dextran and Orgaran.

Dextran 40 (Gentran 40, Rheomacrodex), administered by intravenous infusion, has a molecular weight of about 40 000. *Dextran 70 (Gentran 70, Macrodex)* has a molecular weight of 70 000.

Indications: the solution is used in conditions associated with slow flow and for prophylaxis of postsurgical PE/DVT.

Cautions. Dextrans may interfere with blood group cross-matching or biochemical measurements. They should not be used to maintain plasma volume in situations such as burns or peritonitis where there is a loss of plasma proteins, water and electrolytes over a period of several days. In these situations plasma or plasma proteins should be given. It is necessary to correct dehydration before infusion and give fluids during treatment. Severe congestive heart failure, renal failure, bleeding, thrombocitopenia and hypofibrinogenaemia may occur.

Side effects: rarely, anaphylactoid reaction has been observed.

Dose: by intravenous infusion initially 500–1000 ml, and the subsequent doses according to the patient's conditions.

Orgaran is an antithrombotic, heparinoid drug (mixture of low molecular weight glycosaminoglycuronans including heparan sulphate, dermatan sulphate, and a small amount of condroitin sulphate. This drug is chemically distinct from standard heparin and LMWH. In hip surgery trials it has been used at the dosage of 750 anti-Xa units twice daily subcutaneously. The drug is considered an effective antithrombotic agent in high risk patients for the prevention of DVT, with the potential advantage over unfractionated heparin and LMWH that it does not cross-react with antibodies to heparin or LMWH. The experience so far is limited, as this compound is not widely available.

Other *antithrombotic and heparinoid drugs* are *defibrotide, mesoglycan* and *dermatan sulphate*. However, information about their prophylactic action against DVT and PE is so far very limited.

Drugs Used in Venous Insufficiency

"Venoactive" drugs have been used for symptomatic relief in subjects with venous insufficiency. These drugs (Table 16.2) have very few side effects and are safe. The claimed actions of these compounds are of three types: *symptomatic relief*, improvement of the *venous tone* and decrease of the abnormally increased *capillary permeability and microcirculation alterations, leading to oedema formation*, observed in patients with venous insufficiency. While subjective symptomatic relief has been observed in many patients with venous insufficiency, the claimed action on venous tone has not been clearly documented in humans. The action on the microcirculation and on the increased capillary filtration has been documented in limited studies. Large, double blind prospective studies are needed to confirm whether chronic treatment or chronic prophylaxis with these drugs:

(a) *Used as treatments* — significantly improve signs and symptoms (particularly focusing on oedema);
(b) *Used as prophylaxis* — may affect the evolution of chronic venous insufficiency.

The duration and cost-effectiveness of treatments may also be defined carefully (i.e. in comparison with elastic compression stockings). One important advantage of drug treatment is the possibility of using it in summer or when and where the average temperature is high, as an alternative to compression, which is not well tolerated.

Oxipentiphyllin (Trental) and *Defibrotide (Noravid, Prociclide)* have been used to improve the healing of venous ulcerations in limited prospective studies, with good results.

Oral defibrotide in subjects with chronic venous insufficiency improves the healing time of ulcerations, possibly as a consequence of the profibrinolytic action of the compound.

Oxpentiphyllin possibly improves the healing of venous ulcers by its claimed action on the white cell accumulation in the venous ulcer area.

Table 16.2. Drugs used in venous insufficiency. Only the commercial name and producing company are indicated. This list is incomplete, as several other drugs are available in different countries.

Name	Company
Arvenum 500	Stroder
Venoruton (Paroven)	Zyma/Ciba-Geigy
Centellase	Corvi
Daflon 500	Servier
Doxium 500	OM
Essaven	Rhone-Poluenc/Rorer
Flebosmil	Bouchara
Ginkor	Beaufour
Meliven	Brother
Rutisan CE	Farmitalia
Troxerutin	Negma
Venobiase	Fournier

Drugs Used for Sclerotherapy

Ethanolamine oleate, sodium tetradecylsulphate (STD, Trombovar) and Aethoxysclerol (polidocanol) are used in sclerotherapy of varicose veins. *Phenol* in almond oil is used to treat haemorrhoids.

Cautions: extravasation may cause necrosis of tissue.

Contraindications. Sclerotherapy should not be used in patients with recent DVT, superficial thrombophlebitis, and patients unable to walk. Some authorities suggest avoiding sclerotherapy during treatment with oral contraceptives.

Dose: 2–5 ml of *ethanolamine oleate* (divided between 3–4 sites) are slowly injected in empty, isolated segments of varicose veins.

STD is injected (same procedure) at the dose of 0.1–1 ml into each varicose segment. Up to 4–5 ml can be injected in the same session (see data sheet).

Aethoxysclerol (polidocanol) is used at the concentrations of 0.5%, 1%, 2% and 3%, with the same procedures described before. A very low concentration, according to the experience of the operator, is used in small venous teleangectasias, an increasing concentration in small varicose veins, and higher concentrations (3%) are used only for large varicose veins and perforators.

Elastic compression (bandages and/or stockings) is an essential part of the treatment. *As a simple rule easy to remember, the compression should be maintained at least one week for veins of about 1 mm or less in diameter, at least 2 weeks for veins of about 2 mm, and for at least 3 weeks for veins of 3 mm or more.*

Many other sclerosing agents are available (i.e. *Scleremo* = glycerine chromee and other drugs).

Physical Treatments

Physical treatments of venous and lymphatic diseases are discussed in the relevant chapters. *Leg elevation, increased activity (i.e. walking), physiotherapy (i.e. manual lymph drainage) and weight loss* are all effective measures to be regularly suggested to all patients with venous and lymphatic diseases.

Elastic compression is obtained with stockings or bandages. The two clinical indications for compression are *treatment* of signs and symptoms and *prophylaxis* against the evolution of venous insufficiency and the development of DVT. Compression when used as a treatment significantly improves signs and symptoms (particularly those associated with oedema). When used as a prophylaxis, compression affects the development (reduces the incidence) of DVT and PE and may also affect the evolution of chronic venous insufficiency.

The most important disadvantage of *bandages* is that, to be effective, they have to be carefully placed by an expert (avoiding a tourniquet effect). Also, it is essential to replace them regularly (every 2 or 3 days) to ensure the appropriate compression (and most patients cannot do it by themselves).

Elastic stockings are very effective. They should be tailored to the patient and the problem, but many elderly patients cannot put them on easily.

Graduated compression stockings are mainly used for DVT and PE prophylaxis. Other applications are the postoperative and postsclerotherapy use, as they are more comfortable than bandages.

Pneumatic compression and sequential compression devices (SCDs) are mainly used for DVT and PE prophylaxis. Chronic therapeutic applications include venous ulcerations and lymphoedema. Modified devices are often used for home treatment. The DVT–PE prophylaxis SCDs may also be successfully used.

Local treatment for varicose veins and ulcerations. Most local treatments used for varicose veins, available over the counter in many countries, have not been scientifically tested in prospective studies. The experience in each country is often different in this field. While for varicose veins no local treatment can be seriously recommended, a number of dressings and hydrocolloid dressings have been used in venous ulcerations. However, local treatment may produce severe reactions complicating the clinical problem and must be used with care. In subjects with venous hypertension and eczema, skin protection and hydration may prevent the occurrence of small skin lesions leading to the development of venous ulcerations. When the skin is well hydrated and elastic (i.e. using a neutral skin protector such as Lichtena*), the occurrence of venous ulcerations in the perimalleolar region is greatly reduced.

Note. Treatments, particularly drugs, have different modalities of applications, dosages, and brand names in different countries. Also, many drugs and products used in Europe are not used in the USA and UK, and vice versa. The National Formulary (or the equivalent publication in each country) must always be considered by the reader.

---

*Lichtena A.I.® (UCB) AR-GB11® (furalglucytol)

CHAPTER 17

OTHER VENOUS DISEASES

Athletes' prominent veins may be an occasional clinical problem seen in subjects with hypertrophy of the muscle mass. The decrease in thickness of the subcutaneous tissue makes the veins very prominent. Unless there is serious venous incompetence these veins do not require treatment.

Large dilated or varicose veins in pregnancy appear in some 20% of women below 25 years of age and in a higher percentage (32%) in women above 26. They are only very occasionally a clinical problem. Compression, leg elevation and reassurance are indicated rather than treatment, which is needed only in the case of superficial thrombophlebitis or deep venous thrombosis. Women with large varicose veins or signs of severe deep venous obstruction during pregnancy should receive prophylaxis (i.e. graduated compression stockings and/or low molecular weight heparin prophylaxis before and after delivery). Most veins disappear completely or almost completely within 3–8 months after delivery and any evaluation and treatment of the veins should be postponed (12–18 months) after delivery.

Venous trauma and tumours involving the veins (i.e. the inferior or superior vena cava) occur in a number of patients who usually need complex investigations and prompt treatment. These clinical situations should always be kept in mind as they may occasionally be confused with other causes of venous obstruction (i.e. thrombosis).

Rare Venous Problems

Renal venous thrombosis (RVT) in newborns may most commonly be unilateral or occasionally bilateral. This condition occurs in newborns (over 2/3 of the affected children are under 1 month of age). It may be caused by relative polycythaemia, high vascular resistance or reduced fibrinolysis. Most cases are diagnosed only on postmortem examination. Increased osmolarity associated with hypovolaemia, haemoconcentration and hyperviscosity produces small thrombi in venous radicals and the thrombus formation may progress to the arcuate, interlobular and renal veins. The opposite process is uncommon. RVT causes renal congestion and often infarctions.

The signs and symptoms are a sudden enlargement of one or both kidneys (60%), haematuria, pallor, tachypnoea, vomiting, abdominal distension, shock and oliguria, and finally anuria.

Laboratory findings. Common findings are proteinuria, microangiopathic haemolitic anaemia with red cell fragmentation, thrombocytopenia, low levels of fibrinogen, Factor V and plasminogen and increased concentration of fibrin degradation products. These signs may reflect an active disseminated intravascular coagulation. Urograms cannot be done in this condition. The most useful tests are ultrasound imaging of the kidneys and colour Doppler evaluation of the renal veins and arteries. Isotope renography may also be useful. Venography is risky and usually unnecessary.

Differential diagnosis must be made between RVT and the haemolytic-uremic syndrome. A perirenal haematoma, abscess, hydronephrosis, cysts and tumours may be confused with RVT.

The *treatment* is usually conservative and supportive, aiming to correct the conditions determining RVT. In some cases dialysis is needed. Anticoagulant treatment has been used but its efficacy has not been clearly documented. It may be considered in the case of laboratory findings indicating intravascular coagulation. Surgery is rarely performed. The mortality rate is high and more related to the underlying conditions than to the RVT itself.

The consequences of RVT may be scarring or atrophy of the affected kidney leading to chronic renal failure and, as a late complication, to hypertension. Occasionally kidneys may recover completely.

Renal vein thrombosis in adults is usually a consequence of renal infection, ascending caval thrombosis or caval occlusion due to a tumour thrombus. Treatment should attempt to eliminate the underlying cause. In the case where the diagnosis of unilateral, infective renal vein thrombosis is established, nephrectomy is indicated. In bilateral disease anticoagulant or thrombolytic therapy is indicated.

Rare and Congenital Forms of Venous Anomalies

The *Klippel–Treunaunay syndrome (KTS)* consists of a complex of vascular anomalies usually present at birth which develop further with growth. In early intrauterine life the limb has a ventral vascular system (the primitive femoral artery and veins) and a dorsal or sciatic system. During the second month the femoral develops further while the sciatic system atrophies almost completely. In some subjects the sciatic system persists, generating a large group of venous anomalies included under the name of *KTS* or *lateral venous anomalies*. The arm is affected six times less than the leg. In one out of ten patients the syndrome may be bilateral or affect the upper and lower limb of the same side. Angiomas, varicose veins and hypertrophy in soft tissues and bone prevalently affect the lateral and posterior surface of the limb, often going proximally to the buttock and the vascular territory of the internal iliac artery and vein. According to Dodd and Cockett (1976), three clinical degrees of KTS can be considered:

Type 1 KTS is the fully developed anomaly with skin angioma over the entire, lateral side of the leg from the foot up to the buttock. Deep to the skin and spreading through subcutaneous tissue, muscle and occasionally bone, there is a diffuse angiomatosis. Sometimes the venous spaces flow into the internal iliac vein through a series of large abnormal venous channels. Precapillary AV fistulas may also be present, with increased low resistance arterial flow associated with increased growth of all components of the limb. The leg may be longer and larger. Cases with increased flow at the pelvis causing recurrent rectal haemorrages and very large haemorroids have been also described.

Type 2 KTS is the *pure venous anomaly* with no AV communication and no increase in limb size. Diffuse cavernous haemangioma is the most important feature. It consists of large and small venous spaces well differentiated from large veins which have a well-defined venous wall. There is often a direct communication with the internal iliac vein and often large perforators are observed. A diffuse, patchy capillary haemangioma is present over the lateral and posterior surface of the leg and thigh. Phlebolites and localized thrombi may be observed. Heaviness and disfiguration are the most common complaints. Chronic venous insufficiency may develop if the major incompetent veins are left untreated, and recurrent DVT and PE are possible.

Type 3 KTS is the minor form of the syndrome, presenting as diffuse varicose veins on the lateral side of the thigh and leg. Often no haemangiomas or only small patches are present. Most cases have diffuse, small, tortuous varicosities, usually without evidence of long or short saphenous incompetence.

Diagnosis. The diagnosis is usually clinical. It is possible to evaluate the degree of the vascular anomalies with MRI. Noninvasive investigations (colour duplex and power Doppler) may confirm the presence of an AV communication. Phlebography is used to study the deep veins which may be absent or underdeveloped as their role is taken over by the abnormal veins. Angiography (in the case of diffuse arteriovenous shunting) gives important information and within the same procedure it is sometimes possible to embolize the most important arterial anomalies.

In children it is advisable to investigate the presence of other possible anomalies and to involve the orthopaedic unit because of possible differential growth in the affected limb.

Treatment. In *type 1 KTS* treatment is generally conservative. Patients must be advised to follow a protective policy from a early stage (compression, elevation, avoiding traumas). Most patients benefit from elastic compression. Large incisions in or over haemangiomatous areas may result in chronic ulceration, which are very difficult to heal. Surgery is usually indicated to ligate the larger venous sites or communicating veins or large varices contributing to the chronic increase in venous pressure. When the increase in the growth rate of the limb is excessive, embolization of some of the feeding vessels may be considered. So far there is no standard treatment for this condition, due to the variability of the clinical picture. Surgical treatment should be considered on an individual basis.

Type 2 and 3 KTS are usually managed with compression and selective surgery (often repeated) of the most important venous anomalies. Incisions have to be made on areas of normal skin, as a large incision in an angiomatous area may result in delayed healing. Sclerotherapy whenever possible may help to control the diffuse varicosity. Amputation of the most severely affected limbs has been reported but is now rarely needed.

Prognosis. The variability of signs and symptoms between patients is large. Most patients have a normal, active life. The approach should be optimistic, because conservative treatment and selective surgery are effective in most patients.

Haemangiomas

At a very early stage in the embryo, before arteries, veins and lymphatics become separated as different systems they are organized in systems containing all three vascular elements. Haemangiomas are usually localized congenital vascular malformations with a prevalence of the venous component.

Capillary haemangioma may be superficial or may be part of a more extensive haemangioma situated more deeply. Removal of the lesion is often considered for cosmetic reasons or when the lesion causes repeated bleeding or symptoms. If possible, treatment should be a complete excision of the lesion covering the area with intact skin, as incisions and wounds over haemangiomatous areas heal very slowly.

Cavernous haemangiomas are usually deep masses containing venous spaces which may involve all tissue including bone. MRI reveals the localization and extension of the lesions.

The *diffuse type* is usually treated conservatively, as surgical excision is often impossible. Ligation or sclerotherapy of some venous channels may, however, be beneficial and be considered on an individual basis.

The *localized type* may have a few large venous sinuses which may be successfully removed surgically. However, most lesions appear more localized than they actually are and the surgical field may be more challenging than previously considered. Therefore a careful visualization of the lesion before surgery (MRI, angiography) is essential.

Popliteal Vein Entrapment

Entrapment of the popliteal artery by anomalous anatomy (typically the insertion of the head of the gastrocnemious muscle) causing ischaemic symptoms has been described. The entrapment of the popliteal vein has also been considered as a cause of venous obstruction or a predisposing cause of deep venous thrombosis. The incidence of popliteal vein compression by full knee extension in a normal population has recently been studied by duplex scanning. Knee extension produced complete obstruction in 17% of subjects and severe obstruction (>50% diameter reduction) in a further 10% of subjects. When tested for outflow obstruction, however, only a few limbs revealed an obstruction (by air plethysmography) and less had signs or symptoms of obstruction. The evaluation with phebography of the popliteal vein may show more often a compression which is not clinically relevant. Surgery is very rarely indicated in subjects with signs and symptoms and with documented obstruction.

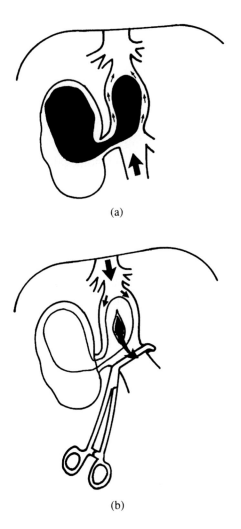

(a)

(b)

Figure 17.1

Renal Adenocarcinoma

The *extension of a renal adenocarcinoma to the inferior vena cava* [Figure 17.1(a)] is due to the growth of the tumour within the venous lumen. In this case the excision of the tumour should be associated with the removal of the neoplastic pseudothrombus [Figure 17.1(b)], which may be below the level of the liver (40%), retrohepatic (45%), or it may reach the right atrium (15%). The treatment required includes caval surgery with complete excision of the tumour and sometimes of the involved caval segment. In some patients cardiopulmonary bypass is necessary.

Splenic Vein Thrombosis

Splenic thrombosis may occur during pancreatitis, in subjects with pancreatic pseudocysts or neoplasm and trauma. Splenomegaly is usually present. Isolated splenic vein thrombosis is a rare cause of variceal bleeding. However, many cases are not associated with bleeding varices and in these patients no treatment is indicated. In other patients splenectomy is indicated.

Splenic and portal problems (portal hypertension, thrombosis) are not discussed in this book, as these problems are usually associated with complex gastro-intestinal and hepatic problems.

CHAPTER 18

THE CEAP CLASSIFICATION

The CEAP classification of venous disorders has been developed by a group of international experts on venous disease with the aim of talking a common language in describing the clinical problems affecting patients.

The meaning of CEAP is:

C = Clinical problems, signs/symptoms
E = Etiology (primary, secondary)
A = Anatomy (sites of venous problems, i.e. in the deep or superficial system)
P = Pathology

The CEAP classification is comparable in aims and structure to the *TNM* classification of tumours and to the *CHAT* classification proposed for cerebrovascular diseases.

So far it has not been widely accepted.

The scoring of venous dysfunctions and disability is presented in Table 18.1. Table 18.2 shows the classification of venous diagnosis.

In an asymptomatic subject with venular dilatations (teleangectasia), the classification according to the CEAP is:

C_1 s.

In asymptomatic subjects with varicose veins the classification is:

C_{2A} EpA_S P_R.

In subjects with an active venous ulceration with incompetence of the long saphenous vein and perforating veins, the classification is:

C_{6S} $EpA_{S,P}$ P_R.

Table 18.1. Scoring of venous dysfunction.

Anatomical Score	**1 Point Each**		SCORE
	Superficial		___
	Deep		___
	Perforator		___
			Subto[ ]

Signs–Symptoms	**0 Points**	**1 Point**	**2 Points**	
Pain	none	moderate, not requiring analgesics	severe, requiring analgesics	
Edema	none	mild/moderate	severe	___
Venous claudication	none	mild/moderate	severe	___
Pigmentation	none	localized	extensive	___
Lipodermatosclerosis	none	localized	extensive	___
Ulcer size	none	<2 cm diameter	>2 cm diameter	___
Ulcer duration	none	<3 months	>3 months	___
Ulcer recurrence	none	once	more than once	___
Ulcer number	none	single	multiple	___
				Subtc[ ]

Disability Score	**0 Points**	**1 Point**	**2 Points**	**3 Points**
	Asymptotic	Symptomatic, can function without support device	Can work 8-hour day *only* with support device	Unable to work even with support device

Subtc[ ]
TOTA[ ]

Table 18.2. Venous diagnosis.

Clinical (C_0–C_6)	Anatomical (A_S, A_D or A_P)
class 0 No visible or palpable signs of venous disease	A_S = **Superficial**
	1 Telangiectases/reticular veins
1 Telangiectases or reticular veins	2 GSV — above knee
2 Varicose veins	3 GSV — below knee
3 Edema	4 LSV
4 Skin changes ascribed to venous disease (e.g. pigmentation, venous eczema, lipodermatosclerosis)	5 Nonsaphenous
	A_D = **Deep**
	6 Inferior vena cava
5 Skin changes as defined above with *healed* ulceration	7 Iliac — common
	8 Iliac — internal
6 Skin changes as defined above with *active* ulceration	9 Iliac — external
Note: The presence or absence of symptoms such as pain or aching denoted by the addition of "S" for symptomatic or "A" for asymptomatic to modify the class category	10 Pelvic — gonadal, broad ligament, others
	11 Femoral — common
	12 Femoral — deep
	13 Femoral — superficial
Etiological (E_C, E_P or E_S)	14 Popliteal
E_C Congenital	15 Crural — anterior tibial, posterior tibial, peroneal (all paired)
E_P Primary, with undetermined cause	16 Muscular — gastrocnemial, soleal, others
E_S Secondary, with known cause — Post-thrombotic, post-traumatic, others	A_P = **Perforating**
	17 Thigh
Pathophysiological (P_R, P_O or $P_{R,O}$)	18 Calf
P_R Reflux	
P_O Obstruction	
$P_{R,O}$ Both reflux and obstruction	

The formulas describing the characteristics of the patient seem more complicated than they really are, and after some experience the classification can be easily applied. It is hoped that it will act as a standard in the reporting of future studies in venous disease and allow direct comparison between different institutions and different treatment methods.

APPENDIX:
FORMS USED IN VENOUS DISEASES

The following two forms are used to indicate superficial incompetence (Form 1) or superficial venous thrombophlebitis, or to indicate the site of deep venous thrombosis, obstruction or incompetence (Form 2).

Form 1: The Superficial System
(Original from S. Hobb's Venous Clinic at St Mary's Hospital, London.)

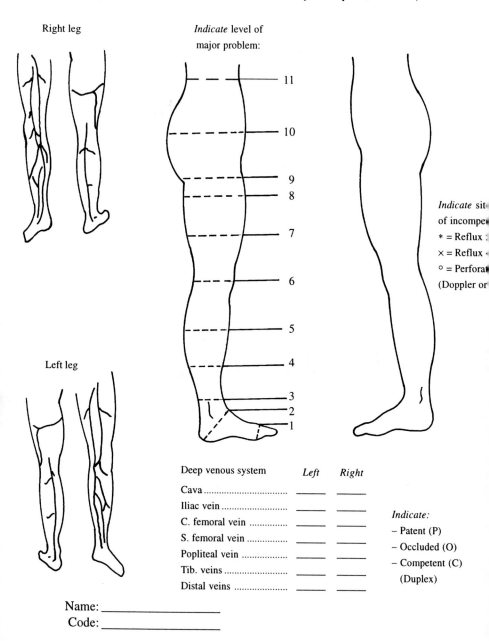

Right leg

Indicate level of major problem:

11
10
9
8
7
6
5
4
3
2
1

Left leg

Indicate site
of incompe...
* = Reflux ...
× = Reflux ...
° = Perfora...
(Doppler or...

Deep venous system	Left	Right
Cava	____	____
Iliac vein	____	____
C. femoral vein	____	____
S. femoral vein	____	____
Popliteal vein	____	____
Tib. veins	____	____
Distal veins	____	____

Indicate:
– Patent (P)
– Occluded (O)
– Competent (C)
  (Duplex)

Name: _____
Code: _____

Form 2: The Deep Venous System

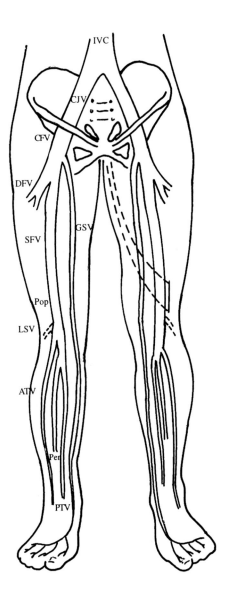

INDEX